P9-DFT-510

THE LOST ART OF CARING

RECENT AND RELATED TITLES FROM
THE JOHNS HOPKINS UNIVERSITY PRESS

John D. Arras, ed.
Bringing the Hospital Home: Ethical and Social Implications of High-Tech Home Care

Robert H. Binstock, Leighton E. Cluff, and Otto von Mering, eds.
The Future of Long-Term Care: Social and Policy Issues

Tom Hickey, Marjorie A. Speers, and Thomas R. Prohaska, eds.
Public Health and Aging

Robert B. Hudson, ed.
The Future of Age-Based Public Policy

Robert Morris, Francis G. Caro, and John E. Hansan
Personal Assistance: The Future of Home Care

Leslie C. Walker, Elizabeth H. Bradley, and Terrie Wetle, eds.
Public and Private Responsibilities in Long-Term Care: Finding the Balance

Carol S. Weisman
Women's Health Care: Activist Traditions and Institutional Change

Carol S. Weissert and William G. Weissert
Governing Health: The Politics of Health Policy

THE LOST ART OF CARING

A Challenge to Health Professionals, Families, Communities, and Society

EDITED BY Leighton E. Cluff, M.D., and
Robert H. Binstock, Ph.D.

THE JOHNS HOPKINS UNIVERSITY PRESS *Baltimore and London*

Printed in the United States of America on acid-free paper
9 8 7 6 5 4 3 2 1

The Johns Hopkins University Press
2715 North Charles Street
Baltimore, Maryland 21218-4363
www.press.jhu.edu

Library of Congress Cataloging-in-Publication Data
The lost art of caring : a challenge to health professionals, families, communities, and society / edited by Leighton E. Cluff and Robert H. Binstock.
p. cm.
Includes bibliographical references and index.
ISBN 0-8018-6591-3 (hardcover : acid-free paper)
1. Care of the sick. 2. Medical care. 3. Nursing home care. 4. Terminal care.
I. Cluff, Leighton E. II. Binstock, Robert H.
RT42 .L67 2001
362.1'023—dc21
00-010271

A catalog record for this book is available from the British Library.

CONTENTS

CONTRIBUTORS

A. E. Benjamin, Ph.D., a professor of social welfare in the School of Public Policy and Social Research at the University of California, Los Angeles, has a background in political science and social work. He has done broad research on long-term services for people with chronic conditions, including the elderly, younger adults with chronic conditions, people with HIV disease, and children with special health needs—particularly issues of comparative access and quality. His recent research has resulted in an edited volume (with Robert J. Newcomer) titled *Indicators of Chronic Health Conditions* (1997) and in various papers and reports.

Robert H. Binstock, Ph.D., a political scientist, is a professor of aging, health, and society at Case Western Reserve University School of Medicine. A former president of the Gerontological Society of America, he has served as director of a White House Task Force on Older Americans and as chair and member of a number of advisory panels to the U.S. government, state and local governments, and foundations. He is the author of about two hundred articles and book chapters, mostly on politics and policies affecting aging. His twenty books include *Home Care Advances: Essential Research and Policy Issues,* coedited with Leighton E. Cluff (2000), and five editions of the *Handbook of Aging and the Social Sciences,* the most recent coedited with Linda K. George (2001). He has received numerous honors and awards in the field of gerontology.

Daniel Callahan, Ph.D., director of international programs for the Hastings Center, was a cofounder of the center and, from 1969 to 1996, its director and president. A visiting scholar at the Harvard Medical School, he is also an honorary faculty member of the Charles University Medical School in Prague. An elected member of the Institute of Medicine, National Academy of Sciences, he was also the recipient of the 1996 Freedom and Responsibility Award of the American Association for the Advancement of Science. He is the author or editor of a number of books, most recently *False Hopes: Why America's Quest for Perfect Health Is a Recipe for Failure* (1998).

Eric J. Cassell, M.D., is a clinical professor of public health at Weill Medical College of Cornell University and an attending physician at the New York–Presbyterian Hospital. He is the author of *The Healer's Art, The Place of the Humanities in Medicine, Changing Values in Medicine, The Nature of Suffering, Talking with Patients,* and, most recently, *Doctoring: The Nature of Primary Care Medicine* (1997). Dr. Cassell is a member of the Institute of Medicine of the National Academy of Sciences, a master of the American College of Physicians, and a fellow and member of the board of directors of the Hastings Center. He currently serves as a member of the President's National Bioethics Advisory Commission.

Leighton E. Cluff, M.D., is immediate past president and trustee emeritus of the Robert Wood Johnson Foundation. He is now a professor emeritus at the University of Florida, where he serves as a member of the University of Florida Health Science Board of Overseers, as an adviser to the University Center on Gerontology, and on the boards of the Institute of Child Health Policy and the Geriatric Center on Graduate Education and Research (Department of Veterans Affairs–Gainesville). A master of the American College of Physicians, Dr. Cluff has published more than two hundred scholarly articles and many book chapters. Among his books are *Helping Shape America's Health Care* (1989), *The Future of Long-Term Care: Social and Policy Issues,* coedited with Robert H. Binstock and Otto von Mering (1996), and *Home Care Advances: Essential Research and Policy Issues,* coedited with Robert H. Binstock (2000).

Nancy J. Cox, M.S.W., is the deputy director of Partners in Caregiving: The Dementia Services Program, in the Department of Psychiatry and Behavioral Medicine at the Wake Forest University School of Medicine. She has been with the National Program Office of this Robert Wood Johnson Foundation project since 1993, becoming responsible for the day-to-day management of the program in 1995. Earlier, she was project director of the Lexington, Kentucky, site in the Dementia Care and Respite Services Program (1988–92), the foundation's predecessor to Partners in Caregiving, and executive director of the Alzheimer's Association in Lexington. She has made presentations at state, national, and international conferences on the topics of Alzheimer disease and adult day programs, and has published in national and international journals.

Claire Fagin, Ph.D., R.N., F.A.A.N., is a consultant to foundations, developing national programs, and educational institutions, and dean and professor emerita of the University of Pennsylvania. She was dean of the School of Nursing at the University of Pennsylvania from 1977 to 1992, and the interim president of the university in 1993 and 1994. Dr. Fagin is a member of the Board of the Radian Group, Inc., the Van Ameringen Foundation, the Visiting Nurse Service of New York, and the New York Academy of Medicine, and is a member or fellow of the Institute of Medicine, National Academy of Sciences, the Expert Panel on Nursing of the World Health Organization, and the American Academy of Arts and Sciences. She has received ten honorary doctoral degrees and numerous alumni, civic, and professional awards. Dr. Fagin has published eight books and monographs and more than seventy-five articles.

Alvan R. Feinstein, M.D., is Sterling Professor of Medicine and Epidemiology at Yale University School of Medicine, where he is director of the Clinical Epidemiology Unit. He is also emeritus director of Yale's Robert Wood Johnson Clinical Scholars Program, in which he is still active as a mentor and teacher. After a research fellowship at Rockefeller Institute, he became medical director at Irvington House, where he studied a large population of patients with rheumatic fever. In this research, he began developing new clinical investigative techniques that were eventually expanded beyond rheumatic fever into his new clinical epidemiologic approaches and methods, which have been reported in three books, *Clinical Judgment*, *Clinical Epidemiology*, and *Clinimetrics*. His clinical orientation to quantitative data has been presented in two other books, *Clinical Biostatistics* and, most recently, *Multivariable Analysis*.

Renée C. Fox, Ph.D., is the Annenberg Professor Emerita of the Social Sciences and a fellow of the Center for Bioethics at the University of

Pennsylvania, where she was professor of sociology, psychiatry, and medicine from 1969 to 1998. She is also a research associate of the University of Oxford. Dr. Fox has lectured widely throughout the United States and Europe on her studies of bioethics, medicine, and sociology. Among her many books are *Experiment Perilous: Physicians and Patients Facing the Unknown* (1959), *Essays in Medical Sociology: Journeys into the Field* (1979), and *The Sociology of Medicine: A Participant-Observer's View* (1989). She is the recipient of many honors and awards, including the Ralph Waldo Emerson Book Award.

Linda K. George, Ph.D., is a professor of sociology and associate director of the Center for the Study of Aging and Human Development at Duke University. She is the author or editor of seven books, more than a hundred journal articles, and more than eighty book chapters. A past president of the Gerontological Society of America and former editor of the Social Sciences section of the *Journal of Gerontology*, she has coedited three editions of *The Handbook of Aging and the Social Sciences.* Her major research interests include social factors and depression; the effects of stress and coping, especially the stress of caring for an impaired family member; the relationship between religion and health; and the effects of beliefs and expectancies on health. Dr. George has received numerous honors and awards for her research and teaching.

Joel D. Howell, M.D., Ph.D., obtained his M.D. from the University of Chicago and his Ph.D. in the history and sociology of science from the University of Pennsylvania. He is now at the University of Michigan, where he is a professor in the Department of Internal Medicine in the Medical School, the Department of History in the College of Literature, Science, and the Arts, and the Department of Health Management and Policy in the School of Public Health. His research focuses on an attempt to understand why and when people in America and England came to believe that technology is valuable for health care.

Kenneth M. Ludmerer, M.D., is a professor of medicine in the School of Medicine and a professor of history in the Faculty of Arts and Sciences at Washington University, St. Louis. His most recent book is *Time to Heal: American Medical Education from the Turn of the Century to the Era of*

Managed Care (1999), which was nominated for a Pulitzer Prize in nonfiction. He is a member of the Association of American Physicians, a fellow of the American Association for the Advancement of Science, and vice president of the American Association for the History of Medicine. In 1997 he received the Nicholas Davies Memorial Award of the American College of Physicians for outstanding contributions to the medical humanities.

Mathy Mezey, Ed.D., R.N., F.A.A.N., has been Independence Foundation Professor of Nursing Education at New York University since 1991, where she is also director of the John A. Hartford Foundation Institute for the Advancement of Geriatric Nursing Practice. Previously, she was a professor at the University of Pennsylvania School of Nursing, where she directed the geriatric nurse practitioner program and the Robert Wood Johnson Foundation Teaching Nursing Home Program. Dr. Mezey's current research focuses on ethical decision making about life-sustaining treatment and decisions related to the transfer of patients between nursing homes and hospitals. She has authored five books and more than fifty articles, and is series editor for the Springer Series in Geriatric Nursing. She was a member of the Ethics Group of Hillary Rodham Clinton's Health Care Reform Task Force.

Burton V. Reifler, M.D., M.P.H., has been professor and chairman of the Department of Psychiatry and Behavioral Medicine at the Wake Forest University School of Medicine since 1987 and is director of the Robert Wood Johnson Foundation's National Demonstration program on Adult Day Services, Partners in Caregiving. Previously, at the University of Washington, he started Geriatric and Family Services, a multidisciplinary outpatient clinic that became a model for the treatment of elderly and Alzheimer patients around the country. A past chairperson of the American Psychiatric Association's Council on Aging, Dr. Reifler has served on numerous national task forces and committees. He has more than one hundred publications and has served on many editorial boards, including his current position as associate editor of the *American Journal of Geriatric Psychiatry.* The 1996 recipient of the Ruth von Behren Award from the National Adult Day Services Association, he was elected to the board of directors of the International Psychogeriatric Association in 1997.

Robyn I. Stone, Dr.P.H., has been executive director of the Policy Research Institute at the American Association of Homes and Services for the Aging since 1999. She is a widely published and internationally noted researcher and authority in the areas of long-term care, chronic care for the disabled, and family caregiving. Dr. Stone served in the Clinton administration as deputy assistant secretary for disability, aging and long-term care policy, and as acting assistant secretary for aging, overseeing the Administration on Aging. She returned to the private sector in 1997, first as a professor of public policy at Georgetown University's Institute for Healthcare Research and Policy and then as executive director of the International Longevity Center in New York City, part of a multinational research and education consortium examining the global implications of population aging.

FOREWORD

THIS book provides a great service by drawing attention to the vital role of caring in health care and caregiving. As it makes clear, caring—the concern, compassion, and support of health professionals, family members, and communities—is of great importance to those who are coping with illness or disability and are in pain and suffering. Effective caring involves meeting not only physical needs but spiritual and psychological needs as well.

Caregiving has been a familiar part of my life since I was twelve years old and my father became terminally ill with leukemia. I was one of four children and, as the oldest and a daughter, my thirty-four-year-old mother depended on me. Since Jimmy and I came home from the White House, we have witnessed firsthand the importance of caring as his mother, brother, and two sisters struggled with terminal cancer. And I helped take care of my mother until she died in 2000 at the age of ninety-four. I have had plenty of opportunities to appreciate the many dimensions of caring.

I have been heavily involved in the field of mental health since my husband was governor of Georgia. From my experiences, I have learned that those taking care of mentally ill family members sometimes become so overwhelmed that they neglect themselves and often become casualties in the process. A sensitive and perceptive discussion in this book portrays the "endless caring" that families provide to loved ones who have severe and persistent mental illness. It also provides an overview of the many other types of illnesses and disabilities that we can experience and the needs for caring that arise from them.

My interest in mental health led to the establishment of the Rosalynn Carter Institute at Georgia Southwestern State University to address the needs of those who give care. We began working with family members of loved ones with mental illness, but our efforts quickly spread to include caregivers for individuals with any kind of illness or disability, including frail elderly persons. Now in its twelfth year, the institute is dedicated to improving the caregiving process. We help professionals and families increase their skills in caring and working harmoniously together. We are now attempting to replicate our programs across the country.

Our experiences at the Rosalynn Carter Institute have led us to build support systems that provide communities of caring for caregivers. We have created CARE-NET, a caregivers' network. Through this network, family and professional caregivers, representatives of local, state, and federal government agencies (social service, mental health, aging, and other), members of religious communities, and advocates all meet together regularly. They discuss the needs of caregivers in our area and try to find solutions to their problems.

Caring for individuals at the end of life is a special concern of mine. As honorary chairperson of the Last Acts Coalition, I join more than five hundred organizations representing major healthcare professional groups, bioethics centers, and consumer and advocacy groups in fostering three major changes: better communication among individuals who are dying, their families, and health professionals; more support for good end-of-life caring from the medical community; and a cultural shift in our society. Most people die in hospitals, often left alone in unrelieved pain, hooked up to machines. As the authors in this book suggest, doctors are taught to heal, and if they cannot, they feel they have failed. We need to change this perception by helping them focus on palliative care—comfort for individuals in the last stages of life.

I strongly commend *The Lost Art of Caring* as essential reading for health care professionals, family caregivers, members of community volunteer organizations, and policy makers. Many circumstances in contemporary society have made caring more difficult now than in the past. This book highlights the challenges to be met if we are to rekindle caring as an essential part of our culture. After all, at one time or another in our lives, we will all need caring.

Rosalynn Carter

PREFACE

It is difficult to appreciate the importance of caring without personally having experienced a serious illness or disability or having had an opportunity to observe close at hand those who are so afflicted. Personal experiences with sickness and disability can have a deep and lasting impact on one's attitudes toward those who are ill or functionally impaired. Books, journals, television, and other media can help one see and sense what it means to be sick, but these are not substitutes for real-life experiences. With medicine's ability to control the manifestations of many acute and chronic diseases, individuals today often have had no significant and personal experience with these problems until they reach advanced age. As Lewis Thomas wrote in 1983 (in *The Youngest Science,* New York: Viking Press: 222), "Most of us can ride almost all the way through life with no experience of real peril, and when it does come, it seems an outrage, a piece of unfairness. We are not used to disease as we used to be."

A few years ago, in a seminar I was conducting for thirty preprofessional college students, a student asked: "Why don't medical schools teach their students how to be compassionate and caring for those who are sick and disabled?" I responded: "If I were to fall out of my chair at this moment with a heart attack, all the compassion, tenderness, and caring you could provide would do me very little good. What I would need is a well-educated and trained physician, who is medically competent; but your attention and concern would be helpful and appreciated if I were to live." Then I asked the students: "Have any of you had an experience in the past few days with a person who was very sick or disabled?" There was a lengthy pause—then a young woman responded: "I think I know what you mean. Yesterday when I was walking across campus, a student using crutches walked toward me. I wondered at the time how he manages to get from one class to another when there is a limited amount of time. How does he feel when classmates are fooling around playing baseball or football or are going to dances? How is he able to relate to girls whom he might like to date or get to know?" At that point, I said: "You have it! Only when you see, feel, attempt to understand, and show concern for another who is sick or disabled can you become a compassionate and caring person. If you have not had such an experience before becoming a medical student, you may never be a caring and compassionate physician."

In 1946, when I was a second-year medical student, a classmate and I developed pulmonary tuberculosis, and we each spent a year in a sanatorium in upstate New York, away from family—and, in my case, away from a wife of just two years. No antituberculous drugs were available then, and bed rest, eating well, and being out of doors in fresh air was the standard treatment. After initial evaluation and reassurance by a physician, I was placed in a cottage with rooms for four patients, two on each side of a living room with a fireplace. I was obliged to sleep on a screened porch outside my room all day and all night. I was up only for toileting. Breakfast, lunch, and dinner were brought by a person driving an exposed pickup truck and were delivered to me on metal-covered plates and trays; I learned to enjoy eggs cooked or uncooked, warm or cold, in any form whatsoever. In the winter, when the temperature on my porch was several degrees below freezing, I slept wearing a ski mask to avoid freezing of my face and usually awoke with frost around my nostrils and mouth. There was no telephone available in the cottage, so it was impossible for me to speak with my wife except on those occasions when I went to the physicians' offices to be examined. However, I received a joyous, humorous, and loving card from her every day (on a Monday, usually two cards). She visited me only four times over almost twelve months, and one of these visits was over Christmas and New Year's, when she did not have to teach (she was a preschool education specialist). During those visits, there were no opportunities for intimacy, and we learned that abstinence can make the heart grow fonder and more eager. Nurses visited me almost every day and provided friendship, kindness, understanding, and caring. They sustained my morale, even when other patients were not doing well (and some died).

During this experience, I came to understand the reality of morbidity and potential mortality. My wife's and my savings for my medical-school expenses were exhausted by payment for sanatorium care, and this made it uncertain as to whether I would be able to return to school. A social worker at the sanatorium, however, watched over all of the patients and tried to meet our "social" and special needs as best she could. When she learned of my problem, she arranged for me to apply for financial support to continue my education. With this assistance, I reentered medical school after a lapse of one year, with my tuberculosis stable, under control, and not contagious; my wife had been regularly tested to determine if I had infected her.

My experience with tuberculosis was not uncommon for medical students before 1950. Only 10 percent of my entering class were tuberculin positive when entering medical school, but almost 80 percent were tuberculin positive on graduation. Only two of us were known to have developed disease from this infection, but infection with the tubercle bacillus was an occupational hazard for medical students before the introduction of streptomycin and isoniazid and the progressive decline in tuberculosis in the United States.

Medical students today do not often develop a serious illness or disability. Many acute and chronic conditions in those who are young now are prevented or cured, or their progress is controlled. Moreover, they are less frequently exposed to serious illnesses in their families when they are young, because most parents and grandparents remain relatively healthy today until advanced old age. Medical students are exposed to serious medical problems, often for the first time, only in the patients they see while in training. But changes in the financing and technology of medical care, particularly in teaching hospitals, have seriously compromised the time and opportunity for medical students to get to know patients as persons; often they see them only as special disease, diagnostic, and treatment problems.

Perhaps it is time for medical schools to provide the time for students, and even interns and residents, to listen to patients who are seriously ill and impaired. This could be done in patient homes, nursing homes, day care centers, institutions for mentally or physically disabled persons, and hospice settings. The short duration of hospitalization for most patients today, and the dominance of diagnostic and therapeutic technology in the hospital, no longer provide suitable experiences for students to appreciate the meaning of serious illness and disability or to understand the need patients have for caring and to be accepted as persons rather than diagnostic and therapeutic problems.

I have observed competent physicians, nurses, and other health care providers who are not caring because of the demands of medical technology and lack of time with patients. When necessary, I have removed a physician from responsibility for a patient's care because of his inability to develop a trusting and supporting relationship with the patient. I have cared for patients who were drug abusers and who have sold illegal drugs to children and I have been perplexed about caring for them. I have seen parents ignore and abuse their sick children, and adults ignore and even abuse their elderly parents. I have witnessed parents caring for their children, adults caring for their aged parents, and spouses and friends caring for each other, even under the most trying and difficult circumstances. My personal experiences with caring for a very old and disabled mother and providing support and caring for many who have been sick, disabled, and dying have contributed to the strength of my belief that caring is as integral a part of medical care and meeting the needs of the sick and disabled as is the availability of advanced medical technology. Moreover, experiences with those who are caring for persons who are very sick or dying convince me that they, too, need understanding, support, and caring from others, including friends, clergy, and particularly health care providers.

These personal experiences strongly influenced my appreciation of the importance of caring for those who are unfortunate or sick and functionally impaired, and that caring can and should be provided by parents, friends, spouse, physicians, nurses, social workers, and every human being. Understanding the needs of sick and disabled persons is important to caring for them. A caring society depends on its members' appreciation of the problems individuals experience when assaulted by serious illness and functional impairment. A few secondary schools and colleges have instituted programs designed to nurture this appreciation by enabling students to visit, listen to, and learn from young and old persons who are sick and impaired at home, in hospitals, nursing homes, mental institutions, and shelters for the homeless and abused. Such efforts are important and should be encouraged if we are to retain a personal, communal, and national spirit of caring.

The idea for this book had its genesis in my thoughts about the importance of caring as a dimension of medical care, as I reflected on my career as a physician and observed contemporary developments in the health care arena. It was nurtured through conversations with several of my physician colleagues, particularly Dick Reynolds. I then drew Bob Binstock into these conversations and, ultimately, into coediting this book, because we had successfully collaborated in the publication of two previous books on related topics: *The Future of Long-Term Care: Social and Policy Issues,* edited by Robert H. Binstock, Leighton E. Cluff, and Otto von Mering (1996); and *Home Care Advances: Essential Research and Policy Issues,* edited by Robert H. Binstock and Leighton E. Cluff (2000).

It is my hope that the essays in this volume on the many aspects and issues associated with caring will provide and encourage a deeper understanding and appreciation of the importance of caring for all who are in need of personal attention and assistance when ill and impaired, by health care providers, families, communities, society, and the nation. The contributors to this book have given much thought and consideration to their chapters, and a prepublication conference provided them with an extraordinary opportunity to share their concern for the future of caring. Perhaps, this book may help everyone respond caringly to those who are sick and disabled.

L.E.C.

ACKNOWLEDGMENTS

WE ARE grateful to the Robert Wood Johnson Foundation for financial support that made possible the preparation of this volume, as well as two previous volumes on which we collaborated. We also wish to thank Shands HealthCare and the College of Medicine of the University of Florida. They provided support for a prepublication conference at which contributors to this volume and a select group of invited guests critiqued draft chapters and discussed the substance of caring.

Wendy Harris, of the Johns Hopkins University Press, provided exceedingly helpful editorial guidance and support throughout this project, which we deeply appreciate. In addition, we want to express our appreciation to Karen Henderson, Jenny Wilson, and Jack Winningham, who provided high-quality and loyal assistance at various stages of this project. We also wish to recognize Beth, Martha, and Jenny for their patience with us during the long days, weeks, and months that it took to bring this work to completion. Finally, we especially want to thank the authors who joined us in this project, both for their splendid contributions and for their patience with our editing.

THE LOST ART OF CARING

INTRODUCTION

> I may be dying, but I am surrounded by loving, caring souls.
>
> Morrie Schwartz, in Mitch Albom's *Tuesdays with Morrie,* 1997

THIS book is about *caring* for persons who are ill, functionally disabled, and/or distressed. Our choice of the term *caring,* as opposed to *care* or *caregiving,* expresses our intent to focus on the humane and palliative aspects of health care that contribute to an individual's quality of life.

Caring comprises a wide range of responses to human vulnerability, frailty, pain, and suffering. Many words can be used to describe its elements—*compassion, comfort, empathy, sympathy, kindness, tenderness, listening, support,* and *being there.* Caring can range from very active efforts to relatively passive attentiveness. Its unifying essence, however, is concern for and responsiveness to the needs and worth of the person receiving it.

Several years ago, a young physician, Dr. Alison Clay, recounted how she came to learn the importance of *caring* as a dimension of medical care. While a medical student, she was suddenly hospitalized in an intensive care unit with severe respiratory difficulty due to an asthmatic episode. As she recalled the experience in a subsequent article in a medical journal:

> I am frightened by the chaos and the number of people required for my care. The seriousness of the situation seems amplified by how systematically everyone is moving: the edge in the physicians' voices as they give orders, the concentration not on me but on the monitors recording my vital signs. I wonder if their silence is a reflection of the seriousness of my condition or just short-sightedness, and assumption that I understand what is happening.
>
> My hypercapnia overwhelms me. The next thing I remember is a

> gentle touch on my forearm, and someone softly telling me where I am, the day and time. I am amazed at how useful this information is to me, how moving the gentle touch, how comforting the kind tone of voice. As a student I feel very self-conscious when I want to reach out and touch a patient. I worry that I will be criticized for not being professional, or mocked for trying to communicate with someone who is obviously comatose. I realize the importance not only of what we communicate but the quality and frequency with which we do it. I wonder if I have ever comforted a patient in this way. How often do I turn my focus from my performance to the needs of the patient? (Clay, 1999: 225–26)

PHYSICIANS AND CARING

Caring has always been integral to medicine's mission. Indeed, in earlier eras, it was often the primary response that a physician could offer to a patient. As Dr. Jacob Bigelow (1852) expressed it in the middle of the nineteenth century, "When we consider that most diseases occupy, from necessity, a period of some days or weeks, that many of them continue for months, and some for years, and finally that a large portion of mankind die of some lingering or chronic disease, we shall see that the study of palliation is not only called for, but really constitutes one of the most common, as well as the most useful and beneficent employments of 'medical care'" (136).

The scientific and technological advances in medicine throughout the second half of the twentieth century greatly enhanced the capacity of physicians to do much more than be caring—to diagnose, treat, and cure, as well as to prevent some diseases and retard the progression of others. And even when an underlying disease or disability cannot be cured or arrested, the power of modern medicine can substantially prolong life and maintain and restore patients' functional capacities and enable them to enjoy a good quality of life. Future advances in the biomedical sciences and technology will undoubtedly be even more remarkable in enhancing what medicine can achieve along these lines. However, attention to caring in the practice of contemporary medicine and the opportunities to undertake it have diminished.

As illustrated by Alison Clay's newfound appreciation of the importance of caring when she was hospitalized while she was an advanced medical student, medical education in recent decades has been heavily concentrated on the scientific and technical dimensions of medicine's mission. Yet, even if this emphasis has been at the cost of attention to the caring aspects of medical practice, one can hardly blame the academic medical establishment. As physician and historian Kenneth Ludmerer (1999) observes in *Time to Heal,* his classic book on U.S. medical education in the twentieth century:

> The power of medical education is limited, particularly regarding its ability to produce doctors who are caring, socially responsible, and capable of behaving as patient advocates in all practice environments. Indeed, much of the behavior of physicians reflects influences from outside the medical school, such as the character and values of those who choose to enter medicine, the cultural climate of the time, and the particular rewards and incentives offered by medical practice. It is important to recognize that the caliber of doctors we have represents a negotiation between medical education and society. Our physicians reflect the type of people and society we are, not just the efforts of academic health centers. (xxi)

Certainly, changes in the organization and financing of health care and the overall ethos of the health care arena have made it more difficult for physicians to give as much emphasis as they might to caring. Starting about two decades ago, the parties that finance most of U.S. health care—government, insurance companies, and large employers who provide health insurance coverage as an employee benefit—became increasingly concerned about the rapidly inflating bills that they paid. Since then they have constantly pressured hospitals and doctors to be more efficient and cost-effective. As a consequence, health care has become more of a "business" than it was in the past. Staff doctors are pressured by administrators to see as many patients as possible. Consequently, they cannot spend as much time with their patients as they did in the past, and therefore are not as able to get to know them as persons—how they cope with sickness and disability; their aspirations, anxieties, and spiritual needs; their occupational, familial, social, and other life circumstances. The growth of prepaid managed care during the past fifteen years has especially accelerated these pressures on physicians.

NURSES AND CARING

Caring has also had deep roots in the nursing profession since its inception in the late nineteenth century. Some years ago, Lewis Thomas

(1983) idealized this role of nurses with his description of how they function in a hospital setting:

> [Nurses] know their patients as unique human beings, and they soon get to know the close relatives and friends. Because of this knowledge, they are quick to sense apprehensions and act on them. The average sick person in a large hospital feels at risk of getting lost, with no identity left beyond a name and a string of numbers on a plastic wristband, in danger always of being whisked off on a litter to the wrong place to have the wrong procedure done, or worse still, not being whisked off at the right time. The attending physician or the house officer, on rounds and usually in a hurry, can murmur a few reassuring words on his way out the door, but it takes a confident, competent, and cheerful nurse, there all day long and in and out of the room on one chore or another through the night, to bolster one's confidence that the situation is indeed manageable and not about to get out of hand. (67)

In hospitals, nursing homes, home care settings, or in a hospice program, there are three dimensions to the caring responsibilities of nurses: patient care, teaching, and advocacy. Patient care, in addition to administering medicines and changing wound and surgical dressings, includes ongoing assessment of and responses to the physical, emotional, and social status of the patient. Teaching is focused on providing patients with adequate knowledge to carry out prescribed regimes, such as taking their medications after discharge from the hospital, and to make a variety of lifestyle choices that can enhance both their recovery from illness and their ongoing health. In their role as patient advocates, nurses attempt to guard against their patients being underserved or inappropriately served by the health care system; for instance, ensuring that a hospital discharge is to an appropriate setting with adequate care.

Even as with physicians, the structures and economics of the contemporary health care scene can make it difficult for nurses to carry out these caring roles. When hospitals downsize their nursing staffs in order to reduce costs, the efforts of those nurses who remain tend to be spread thin. They have less time to spend with their patients and for getting to know them so that they can carry out their nursing care, teaching, and advocacy roles. Similarly, the economics of the home care industry today rarely allow for visiting nurses to spend enough time with their patients to establish a caring relationship.

CARING BY FAMILIES AND COMMUNITY ORGANIZATIONS

From the dawn of human history, of course, families—parents, grandparents, children, siblings, and extended kin—have been the major source of caring for their sick and disabled relatives. And this remains true today, despite the proliferation of hospitals, nursing homes, assisted-living and board-and-care facilities, group homes, home care services, and many other health care institutions and programs.

Yet, in contemporary society, many factors contribute to the attenuation of family caring. More families are geographically dispersed than in the past; retired parents migrate to new locales and adult children settle in communities other than those in which they grew up. Sustained high rates of divorce and out-of-wedlock births have created more situations in which a single parent is confronted with the competing pressures of caring for a child and maintaining essential income from employment. The same dilemma is experienced by an increasing number of households in which it is necessary for two parents to work in order to secure sufficient income.

When persons who have no family need caring or (for one reason or another) family members are unavailable for caring, voluntary community organizations—sectarian and nonsectarian—have helped to fill the breach throughout most of American history. Their wide variety of efforts range from the establishment of nursing homes and other venues for care of the sick and disabled, through the provision of food and shelter, to counseling and emotional support. Especially notable in recent times has been the development of support groups, organized around specific illnesses and disabilities; for example, heart disease, cancer, and spinal-cord injury. In addition to being a venue for the exchange of medical information, these support groups are highly focused on the nonmedical aspects of caring, enabling ill, recovering, and disabled participants to share with each other their anxieties and frustrations, as well as practical advice regarding their day-to-day activities and long-term prospects and aspirations. Some of these groups—such as those organized around Alzheimer disease, severe and persistent mental illness, and mental retardation—are primarily oriented toward caring family members, to help them deal with the ongoing stresses that they experience.

SOCIETY AND CARING

Caring is also undertaken by American society through governmental actions, though in a very different dimension than the caring provided by doctors, nurses, families, and voluntary organizations. Despite a political tradition that generally militates against government intervention, the public sector does a great deal to promote the health of Americans—through public health programs; regulation of health care services, health-related products, and health insurance; financing biomedical research and the training of health care professionals; and funding health care for selected segments of the population.

There are many gaps in societal caring, however, and two among them are particularly notable as we begin the twenty-first century. One is the absence of health insurance for 16.3 percent of the U.S. population (U.S. Census Bureau, 1999), which substantially impedes their access to health care. The other is the inability of middle-class families to pay for the very high costs of long-term care in nursing homes or in home- and community-based settings when family members are not available to be caregivers. This latter gap will be exacerbated considerably in the decades immediately ahead because the baby-boom cohort will be entering old age, a time of life characterized by high rates of functional dependency.

PURPOSES OF THIS VOLUME

The purposes of this book are to draw increased attention to the integral role of caring in health care, as well as to contemporary forces that seem to downgrade caring or make it difficult to undertake. Its intended audiences are health care professionals and students; administrators of health care institutions and programs; family members, members of voluntary organizations, and other laypersons who provide care and caregiving for relatives, friends, and strangers; and policymakers concerned with shaping American society to be humane and caring.

The opening part of the volume discusses the nature and meaning of caring and the populations that require it. Daniel Callahan explores the many dimensions of our need for caring and the types of caring that can be provided. A. E. Benjamin and Leighton E. Cluff provide an overview of the many types of illnesses and disabilities that we can experience and the needs for caring that arise from them. Burton V. Reifler and Nancy J. Cox treat particular issues that arise in caring for persons with severe and persistent mental illness, especially the challenges faced by family members.

The provision of caring is discussed in the six chapters of part II. Joel D. Howell presents a history of caring by families, physicians, and nurses in the United States, from colonial days through the twentieth century. Eric J. Cassell analyzes contemporary factors that bear on the capacity of physicians to be caring. Kenneth M. Ludmerer and Renée C. Fox address the erosion of caring in medical education due to the commercialized culture of contemporary academic health centers. Mathy Mezey and Claire Fagin examine caring as it is provided in hospitals and nursing homes, with particular attention to the role of nurses. Robyn I. Stone delineates a number of challenges involved in caring as it takes place in home- and community-based settings by family members and health care professionals, as well as relevant policy issues. And Linda K. George presents an analysis of the strengths and limitations of various types of voluntary organizations as they endeavor to be caring.

The two chapters in part III deal with evaluation of caring, but from quite different perspectives. Building on a critical review of concepts and methods used to measure the quality of medical care, Alvan R. Feinstein proposes a new approach for appraising the success of caring. Robert H. Binstock addresses the question of whether society is caring with respect to the health of its people, as expressed through governmental actions and inactions.

At the end of the book, a summary presents the main points made in earlier chapters.

REFERENCES

Albom, M. (1997). *Tuesdays with Morrie: An Old Man, a Young Man, and Life's Greatest Lesson.* New York: Doubleday.

Bigelow, J. (1852). In Robert Coope, ed., *The Quiet Art: A Doctor's Anthology,* p. 136. London: Livingstone.

Clay, A. (1999). The medical student as patient. *Annals of Internal Medicine* 131(3), 225–26.

Ludmerer, K. M. (1999). *Time to Heal: American Medical Education from the Turn of the Century to the Era of Managed Care.* New York: Oxford University Press.

Thomas, L. (1983). *The Youngest Science.* New York: Viking Press.

U.S. Census Bureau (1999). *Health Insurance Coverage: 1998.* Current Population Survey, P60-208, October.

I

CARING AND THE POPULATIONS IN NEED OF IT

1

Our Need for Caring

Vulnerability and Illness

DANIEL CALLAHAN, PH.D.

RECALL the old children's game, "What's wrong with this picture?"

I am asked by a conscientious physician, a friend in charge of an intensive care unit, to spend some time talking about ethics with his staff. We begin the day with rounds, the usual small group of residents and medical students going from patient to patient. As an outsider I stand back from the group, watching them with interest. They come to one critically ill patient, an elderly woman. They circle about the monitors, intent on understanding the patient's condition, talking quietly about what the dials and screens reveal.

My friend says a word to the patient, who is fully conscious, but only a word. He is the only one who looks at her. Her face shows considerable anxiety. No one appears to notice. Machines, it seems to be understood, tell more about a patient's condition than faces. As this picture unfolds, an elderly man approaches the group. No one notices him, but it seems evident that he is the husband of the patient, and—if attention is paid to his face—a *worried* husband. Somebody, it seems, should speak to him. Anybody. So I do. The man leaves . . . my unofficial response, saying that I, too, am a visitor, having seemed not quite adequate.

The rounding group moves on to the next patient. We later discuss some ethical problems perceived by the staff. I said nothing about the way the group interacted with the patient since it was caught up in an analysis of other issues. But I should have spoken up; there was something terribly wrong with that picture, and almost as wrong as another picture I recalled at that time. Two days before my mother's death, her long-time family physician came to visit her in the hospital. My stepfather and I were there and my mother was fully conscious, perfectly able to talk. Her doctor chatted with us for twenty minutes without once looking at her, even as he was leaving the room. That time I was astonished. It was a stunning act of insensitivity—although that word is too mild to use in describing the event.

Does that matter? The patient I saw in the intensive care unit was receiving technically superior care, as was my mother. Isn't that what counts? Not quite. At the heart of the medical enterprise lies a powerful drive: to relieve our pain and suffering and to reduce our biological vulnerability to decline and decay. This drive is responsible in great part for the enormous improvements in life expectancy and health that were a signal mark of the twentieth century. Along with the democratic ideal of the individual's necessary role in shaping our public social and political life, and the moral goal of self-determination in our private life, the medical drive to improve our often-precarious biological life is understood as part of a larger vision of human progress.

Yet it is a vision that is ambivalent about the permanent need for human caring. From even a casual glance at our biological history, it is easy to see that human life began as fragile and constantly threatened and for most of human history continued that way. Illness and death were ever-present realities, joining the man-made threats of war and social violence as constant reminders of the inescapable precariousness of the human condition. That situation in turn gave rise to the perceived need for humans to care for one another, not only physically but also spiritually and psychologically. Children could not survive if they were not cared for. Comforting hands had to be laid on the sick to relieve pain, and collective meaning had to be constructed to make sense of the seeming fragility of life. It was thus easy, because so obviously necessary, for ancient and premodern medicine to give a primacy to caring—by which I will mean, in a preliminary way, being with a patient emotionally and cognitively, sensitive to the patient's need, devoted to the patient's welfare. There was hardly any other choice, no other plausible ideal.

Modern medicine has single-mindedly pursued an alternative ideal, and herein enters the ambivalence. Its aim is not only to relieve pain and suffering, and to forestall death, traditional enough goals. It also aims, in its practices and proclivities, to help us as individuals to transcend the need for caring, to minimize our biological vulnerability, and to allow us to use medical skills to pursue our own values and ways of life. The modal creature of contemporary life, celebrated in our media and advertising, is the healthy, fit young adult, footloose and fancy free, or the well-preserved, vital senior citizen; each of them is shaping a fast-paced life of unlimited horizons and unimpeded self-direction. Medicine is supposed to give us the body to do that, while both the market and good government are providing the sustaining economic and social environment.

Under such a popular scenario, caring, as a value, can be downgraded, delisted, maybe someday eliminated, in that best of all possible worlds. Who will need it? Not the young, who with adequate parental care will survive infancy and who will see genetic disease and childhood cancers vanquished. Not the old, who will have longer lives and, through the magic of technology, healthier lives, lives of travel and fresh self-discovery on the golf course or in mastery of the internet.

There is a problem with those fantasies. They are unreal; or, better, they take a half-truth and turn it into the full truth. Vulnerability is never conquered; it is only kept at bay for a time. Caring is not needed when it is not needed. But even in these heady days of medical progress, the great cures (as always) lie just over the next hill—tomorrow, or maybe next year, whatever and whenever. Only the luckiest of lives will end without a need for caring at some point or other, and almost certainly at the end. The essence of our vulnerability is that, modern medicine or not, we can still be struck down at any time in our lives, through accident, misadventure, or the still-unconquered diseases that fill the pages of the latest medical textbooks and manage to keep our hospitals busy.

Worse still, because therapeutic medicine is exceedingly proficient at keeping us alive when we should be dead, or of sustaining us with one prop or another when we are disabled, or giving us new drug upon new drug to calm our nerves or relieve our anxieties, the need for caring can last for historically unprecedented long periods of our lives. That is exactly what it means to have a chronic disease, not curable but manageable. And there are enough of those diseases to nicely go around, almost guaranteeing each of us at least one of them before we die.

In short, while the dreams of modern medicine have us transcending vulnerability and the need for caring, the old-fashioned reality is still with us, and will always be with us. To be cared for by others, to need caring, remains a permanent part of the human condition. The drive for medical cures, the hype of research agendas, the classy ads of glowing elders on their way to see the Galapagos Islands, Viagra at the ready, serve only to mask that permanence. More than that, they have managed to make caring seem like a second-rate activity, something we do for the biological losers, something we try to hide from public view, something we hire the poor and near-poor to relieve us of at the minimal wage level, or the females in our families, who are expected to do it for nothing.

THE NEED FOR CARING

But why, exactly, do we need caring? And why should it never, not ever, be put in a second-class position? To begin answering those questions, let me return to the theme of human vulnerability. The great contribution of the Enlightenment to medicine was that it set out to do great things for the human condition—most notably, to relieve suffering, the very stuff of flawed biological life. Suffering became an evil not to be understood and accommodated but to be eliminated. Karl Marx once said that the task of philosophy is not to understand life but to change it. For its part, scientific medicine seems to have said that it is not its task to understand and give meaning to suffering but to rid our lives of it. Meaning, like caring, is for the losers.

As it turns out, suffering is still with us and people still try to find meaning. Even if there is no physical pain or disability, sickness can produce misery and despair, calling out for some redeeming sense and purpose, often not found. Caring is needed in order that we can help each other bear the assaults upon order and rationality that disease brings, destroying, or threatening to destroy, the orderly world of customary good health, so invisible when we have it, so wrenching and all-consuming when it is absent.

If it is the loss of a sense of wholeness and bodily integrity that is at the heart of illness and thus at the center of our need for caring, the manifestations of that loss can be many, beginning with a threat to the way we have understood our lives. But if that is perhaps the ultimate threat of illness and disability, it is hardly the only one. The body can experience pain. The body can fall apart. The body can become crippled and disabled, or frail and inadequate, not up to the ordinary tasks of life. The body can lose its vital capacities, for vision and hearing and balance and strength. If such threats are severe enough, we may need the active physical assistance of others and be unable to function without it. If the loss of capacity is less threatening, we may nonetheless require some assistance from others in order that we can remain independent, able most of the time to care for ourselves.

Yet, sometimes we can function well enough, or put up with the pain, or drag our bodies about on our own, and still be needy. We may need simply the presence of others, to keep us from turning dangerously inward with self-pity; or the empathy of others, to help us know that our situation is a concern of others—that they understand what we are going through and want to provide moral and psychological strength for our otherwise private struggle. It is often the seemingly trivial, unnoticed features of life—the casual touch of others, the quiet companionship that friendship brings, the look of concern on the face of a nurse—that constitute the day-to-day security of our lives. Illness and disability can destroy them and only caring can help reconstitute them, bringing back into our lives not only the familiarity of ingrained routine that helps give meaning, but also the presence of others, restoring community and banishing loneliness and isolation.

PARADOXES OF CARING

I have so far done no more than point out the commonest circumstances in which our vulnerability calls forth, or should call forth, a response of caring: when we need meaning, when our bodies need help, and when our psychological or spiritual suffering calls for empathy and understanding. But there is also a somewhat different way of understanding the need for caring, which I will call the paradoxes of caring: to care for patients in order that they may see their condition improved, but knowing all the while that with some patients it cannot be improved and that at some point in every life everything will come to an end.

From one perspective, it can be said that sick and disabled people need caring in order that, despite their condition, their lives can be brought back to normal. Here one begins with those conditions of life thought most conducive to human welfare, seeking to approximate them as much as possible. They include the maximization of functioning, mentally and physically, the prevention of dependency and the pursuit of autonomy, the relief of pain and suffering, a sense of physical and psychological security, and the realization of psychological and spiritual needs. But what happens when that positive mission fails or at least cannot succeed in any significant way? At that point, some different values and stances must be brought to bear, and they can be in tension with the more therapeutic mission—calling it into question, requiring a different response.

The Maximization of Functioning

The ability to carry out what are known professionally as the activities of daily living is one simple standard of good health. If we can feed ourselves, take care of our own toileting demands, move about safely, and get where we have to go, then we have maximized our basic functioning. Curative medicine takes as its goal giving us back that capacity if illness has robbed us of it. But if it cannot do so, then something else is needed. How can a patient learn to function in some partial way if functioning cannot be maximized? Physical help and rehabilitation may do the job. But what if the course is entirely downhill, the capacity to function at the level of daily living steadily declining? Then the need for caring becomes all the more acute. There is no going back to normality, and even rehabilitation is a lost dream. Here is where caring really matters: when nothing that is thought of as a fruit of modern medicine can be applied with any success. Only direct physical help, the constant presence of another, and the steady nourishment of empathy will suffice to help the patient make it through life.

The Prevention of Dependency and the Pursuit of Autonomy

Hardly any cultural value in our society has a higher standing than the pursuit of autonomy and the avoidance of dependency. My mother, who was born in 1895, said constantly to me, "I don't want to be a burden on my children." *Her* mother, ill and failing, had moved in with my parents when they were newlyweds, coming close to ruining their early years together. It was hardly surprising that my mother did not want to repeat that disaster. Yet there was more there: she had imbibed, as we all have, the notion that the individual should be in control of his or her life. We are supposed to manage our own lives, to choose our own destinies, to get out from under the thumb of others or the need for care by others. A high goal of medicine is to make that possible, giving us the physical and mental wherewithal to have a good chance of managing life on our own. We are meant to be neither a burden on ourselves nor a burden on others. And medicine often does a superb job in making that possible.

But not always. Sometimes it does not work and, like it or not, we become dependent, our autonomy severely compromised or lost. Then there are two problems to be dealt with. One of them is that of caring for a patient who has lost autonomy and is dependent upon others. That takes particular skills, most of them demanding, and most centered on physical care. The other problem is that the patient has been put into that culturally most dreaded situation—a state of dependency, lacking autonomy. A large percentage of those who chose physician-assisted suicide (PAS) in Oregon, the one state where it is legal, were not people suffering from any worse physical pain than others. Nor were they less functional than others with similar medical conditions. And most were in hospice programs. It was the loss of their autonomy and the control of their lives that pushed them to PAS (Chin et al., 1999).

Apart from the most extreme cases, those for whom no degree of comfort or caring will relieve them of their sense of existential loss of self-control, the challenge of caring will be to show that there is no inherent loss of human dignity in dependence upon others, and that lives can be well lived even if autonomy is absent. But that kind of message can be delivered only by someone who already has that understanding. It is our culture that instills such notions about an autonomous self, absent in many other cultures. Caring in this case requires caring for people who are dependent in such a way that their condition is shown to be irrelevant to their worth in the eyes of others. More than empathy is required; it is more like helping to convey a different way of thinking about the worth of a life.

The Relief of Pain and Suffering

What could be more central to the great traditions of medicine than the relief of pain and suffering? Only in recent years, however, in great part due to the work of Dr. Eric Cassell, has a sufficiently sharp distinction been drawn between pain and suffering. Pain, ordinarily associated with extreme physical discomfort and distress, is not the same as suffering, commonly identified with psychological or spiritual travail (Cassell, 1991). One can be in pain but not be suffering, and suffer but not be in pain. Ordinarily, the relief of pain can be accomplished with good pharmaceuticals and the necessary skills in using them. It is not, to be sure, always easy to identify with the pain felt by another and there are also considerable variations in what both patients and physicians consider tolerable levels of pain. Even so, skilled clinicians should be able to find ways to identify serious pain in others and take into account, as well, their own values concerning the enduring of pain. The skills necessary to treat suffering—most often, talk and the comforting presence of a health care worker—can be more demanding, but such a course is open to the sensitive clinician.

Not all pain and suffering can be relieved, however, and it is just this recognition that has fueled the recent drive for physician-assisted suicide. That is not an issue I want to take up here, other than to say I oppose it (see Callahan, 1993). More pertinent is the seeming inadequacy of caring when all other avenues of relieving suffering have failed and are likely to continue failing. Some twelve of the fifteen people to request PAS during its first year in Oregon were in hospice programs, and there is no reason to believe that there was some special inadequacy in their caring. Caring, in a word, can fail, or at least encounter some patients who seem indifferent to it and unresponsive to it. I would argue, however, that caring ought to be provided whether it "works" or not. Practical success is not its proper measure. It is what we give to people because they are people, trying to tailor it to their particular needs. It is better if it succeeds, and is in some way helpful, but nonetheless it should always be provided as a measure of respect for the other person, a way of recognizing their humanity and our shared human condition. Better if it is efficacious, but good and imperative even if it is not.

Physical and Psychological Security

Serious illness and deadly diseases first attack our bodies and then, with that work done, rob us of our sense of security in the world. Everything comes crashing down and, in that circumstance, we are doomed to seeing at least the world of our body and our health fall apart. One of the first tasks of caring is to help a person deal with the perception that bodily integrity has been lost and, perhaps in its wake, the integrity of the self as well; selves and bodies cannot be wholly distinguished. This is often possible, for a good deal of caring is to provide support, sympathy, and understanding, as the patient works through to a new integration.

The self, at first threatened in what seems a hopeless way, can reintegrate itself, learning to cope with a different kind of body, one less friendly and familiar than earlier, but a body with which a wary truce can be worked out, one sufficient to allow life to go on. A fundamental contribution of caring is to help patients through that hopeless phase, giving them initially, and in a vicarious way, sufficient psychological props and reassurance that they can begin moving on their own into the new world they must now inhabit. In the case of acute illness, it may be a temporary world. In the case of chronic illness, it may be the world they will have to live in for the rest of their life. Good caring can help people make that transition, the kind of caring that understands it is not just pain or disability at stake but a change in self-understanding and one's place in the physical and social world.

Yet once again caring may not always work, much as the attempt to relieve pain and suffering can fail. This seems particularly true with patients who have a fixed view of themselves—the young athlete who cannot imagine his body not allowing him to participate in sports, the well-ripened, mature adult who cannot give up jogging (that's me), the elderly person, once physically proficient, who must now use a walker. Caring in those circumstances—I have gathered this from experience—has a difficult task. We might well believe that such people have an exceedingly narrow notion of their own talents and possibilities, which is probably true, but not only they but their caretakers as well are stuck with it. While I think it perfectly appropriate—indeed, that it be a demand of serious caring—to engage such people in serious dialogue, if not debate, we may fail. We may know that they are making a mistake, that there are other possibilities in their lives. Even so, caring is needed, if only to help people cope with what might be their misperceptions of life and its possibilities.

Realizing Psychological and Spiritual Needs

Good and effective caring must extend into the psychological and spiritual life of patients. For the seriously ill patient in particular, the shattering of the sense of physical security that is the mark of good health can be a great shock. It affects not only the body but also the self—that self that must make sense of the world. If the aim of the caregiver should be, so far as possible, to restore the body to its original healthy state, it no less should be to restore the patient's spirit to its original state. If that cannot be accomplished, then an urgent task for the caregiver will be to help the patient live with the new situation, and help the patient to fashion a new self that has the strength and integrity to do so. Of course there is, strictly speaking, no "new" self, but rather a self that has resituated itself in the world and in relationship to itself. Here we might think of the caregiver as a kind of midwife, helping the patient bring to birth the self of the future.

Sometimes that will not be possible, no matter how supportive and insightful the caregiver. Some people despair: they cannot imagine living with a body that is different from the one with which they grew up; nor can they imagine finding a way to reconstitute the self to allow it to make sense of, and at least acquiesce in, its new situation. The caregiver may be quite helpless at that point, unable to give the patient what is so desperately needed: new meaning and new purpose. But as in other situations where nothing can be done, caring is still needed. No one wants to be abandoned, even if nothing can be done for them. Indeed, a person who is in despair needs someone with them, just to help them bear it. Moreover, room must be left for the possibility that the darkness will lift, the despair will lessen. That is far less likely to happen, however, if caring has been denied or seriously diminished.

LEVELS OF CARING

By speaking of the paradoxes of caring, I have tried to invoke a feel for the tensions of caring, where the possibility of improving the patient's condition by caring must, realistically, be open to failure. Or better, perhaps, where the need for caring on the part of a patient shifts from being nurtured back to health to the need to be sustained in the face of a failure to achieve that goal. Caring must, in a word, be understood as something people *always* need, when it can help them become better off and when it can perhaps do no more than keep them from total collapse, physical or psychological, as the case may be.

Caring can most usefully be understood at the level of the general and the particular. By speaking of "the general," I mean those cross-cutting forms of caring that are almost always needed by patients, whatever their condition and whatever the situation of the caregiver. By "the particular" I refer to that critical mode of caring that works to understand this patient at this time in this circumstance, seeking to find what is unique about the patient and his or her needs.

The General Levels of Caring

I believe it is appropriate to distinguish at least four levels of general care, which I contend are necessary for all patients, even if there is no expressed desire for the care or even any apparent reason for it at first blush. There is the *cognitive* level, where the need of a person is to have others grasp how he thinks, the way his mind works. This is an often-neglected feature of caring, if only because caring is most commonly thought of as addressing the emotional needs of patients. But our thinking affects our emotions and, in any case, quite apart from the emotions, understanding a sick person's train of thought, how they rationally frame their life and the problems it presents, is crucial. The person in need of caring has a mind, and that mind needs to be addressed. Speaking the truth, articulating the nature of the illness suffered by a patient, laying out the prognosis—all these bear on the kind of caring that addresses our nature as rational beings.

There is the obvious level of *feeling and emotion,* where the threat of illness to the patient's sense of integrity is translated into fear, anxiety, dread, or depression. *Suffering* is a word that can encompass the emotion of meaninglessness, where judgment and feeling merge, or at least seem to; or where the persistence of pain that cannot be fully relieved elicits dread of the future, which promises to bring more of the same. Caring must address the emotions, and *empathy* is the characteristic term chosen to convey the need for those who do the caring to share, even if in an attenuated way, the emotion of the one being cared for. Caring entails a drawing out of oneself, an identification with what the other person is going through, a joining of feeling with feeling.

To the levels of the cognitive and the emotional, I would add a level of *values.* Caring requires an understanding of what the stricken or suffering person values in life. That may encompass those goals and commitments that people have in the way they live their lives, what they cherish in their life. It may require grasping what another person might perceive as an evil in her life, or what would constitute in her eyes an unforgivable failure, or what would be considered a dangerous diminishment of qualities and traits she may have cultivated. It may well be that the values of the suffering person are wrong, or narcissistic, or trivial. That does not matter. For the caregiver they must be understood and worked with, perhaps even to the point of wrestling with another to see if some self-destructive values or mistaken self-perceptions can be changed before it is too late.

The final level might best be called the *relational.* How does a person in need of care and caring see relationships with other people? For some people, life with others is easy and open, marked by friendliness and curiosity about others. But there are many people who do not so easily respond to others—those we think of as distant, or self-contained, or withdrawn, for whom life with others seems more a burden than a pleasure. Trying to grasp where a person falls along the spectrum of possible relationships with others is crucial, if only because the caring can be misplaced, or beside the point, or, worse still, understood wrongly. Good caring works to see how people interact with and relate to each other. The person providing the caring has to determine just what kind of person is the recipient of the caring—that person with whom the caregiver will work to establish a healing, or helping, or consoling, or affectionate bond.

In speaking of the general levels of caring, I have tried to incorporate the different levels with which we as individuals encounter life: with the mind, with feelings, with values, and in relationships with others. There is a considerable literature on the problem and nature of caring, but it often leaves unclear whether caring should be considered a goal-oriented activity, aiming for a particular outcome, or a set of virtuous traits in caregivers, or a type of relationship of one person to another (Allmark, 1995; Morse et al., 1990; Veatch, 1998). I believe that caring, to be meaningful, must have a goal, both general in nature, bearing on what we need as human beings, and particular, bestowing what we need as individuals. If we are treated only as needy human beings, independent of our particularity, the caring may fail. We will not get what we particularly need. Yet if only our particularity is addressed, our sharing in the human condition may be slighted. One way or another, however, caring cannot be unguided, without goals. Otherwise it is likely to miss its mark, not giving us what we need; and that, after all, is the point of caring. But the importance of a goal for caring comes out most strikingly when the particularity of a patient calls forth the caring, when we try to understand what kind of caring a patient needs and the caregiver then seeks to provide.

The Particularity of Caring

I can do no better to bring out this point than to cite some passages from writers who have caught, far better than I have, what might be called the particularity of caring. I begin with a passage from Tolstoy's masterpiece *The Death of Ivan Ilych,* a story not only about the coming of death but of the failure of those around Ivan to give him what he needs:

> What tormented Ivan Ilych most was the deception, the lie, which for some reason they all accepted, that he was not dying but was simply ill, that he only need keep quiet and undergo a treatment and then something very good would result. . . . This deception tortured him—their not wishing to admit what they all knew and what he knew. . . . The awful, terrible act of his dying was, he could see, reduced by those about him to the level of a casual, unpleasant, and almost indecorous incident . . . and this was done by that very decorum which he had served all his life long. He saw that no one felt for him, because no one even wished to grasp his position. (Tolstoy, 1960: 137)

This passage hardly requires an interpretation: I would simply note how brilliantly Tolstoy underscores part of the essence of caring—the need to have one's position grasped. This takes imagination, empathy, and what Ivan most wants—a willingness of others to accept the truth.

In his essay "Imelda," the surgeon Richard Selzer gives us a different kind of caring, this time coming from a distinguished surgeon known for telling the truth to his patients: "With the patients he was forthright. All the facts laid out, every question anticipated and answered with specific information. He delivered good news and bad with the same dispassion" (Selzer, 1995: 255). In a case that Selzer recounts, the surgeon loses on the operating table a young girl about to undergo a procedure to repair a terrible cleft lip and palate. Knowing the importance of the operation to the girl's mother, who could accept the death of her child but not the thought of the child entering heaven with such a terrible disfigurement, the surgeon later returns to the corpse and repairs the lip and palate. The child is, finally, lovely, though in death, the mother satisfied.

Dr. Selzer wishes that he had told the surgeon what it took him some time to see—"that his unrealistic act was one of goodness, one of those small, persevering acts done, perhaps, to ward off madness. Like lighting a lamp, boiling water for tea, washing a shirt" (Selzer, 1995: 262). Caring, I would say, extends beyond a patient to that patient's family, and can extend no less to someone who is dead, someone seemingly beyond caring but whose needs can still be honored; and it can be provided by someone who, by all appearances, lacks precisely those virtues we associate with caring—the warm, giving, sympathetic person. All it takes is an act of goodness.

Finally, I cite a splendid passage by the sociologist Arthur Frank about his own deadly illnesses, a heart attack followed almost immediately by cancer, and about the kind of caring he thinks most important:

> Most people who deal with ill persons do not want to recognize differences and particularities because sorting them out takes time. Even to learn what the differences are, you have to become involved. Generalities save time. Placing people in categories, the fewer the better, is efficient; each category indicates a common treatment: one size fits all. But . . . treatment is not care. Treatment gets away with making a compromise between efficiency and care by creating an illusion of involvement. . . . What makes an experience real is particulars. One person's anger or grief may differ so much from another's that calling them by a common name only obscures what is actually going on for each. . . . It takes time for an ill person to understand her needs . . . [and] being critically ill means never being able to keep up with your own needs. (Frank, 1991: 45–46)

By his emphasis on particularity, Frank says what most needs to be said about caring: that it is caring for this person at this time with this condition in this social or family situation. He also notes a point often overlooked: that while the ill need caring, they may not themselves know what kind of caring. Thus we are forced back to an important insight about caring. There are many ways of caring, and many ways in which patients need caring. A smile may give the patient what he needs, just as a touch may do so. But then again, that may not do it.

We need to know just what it is a patient most needs and what it is, in our relationship to that person, in us to give. That is a heavy demand, one that a casual use of the term *caring*, common enough these days, does not quite capture. It can be easier than most people think, some of the time, but also, some of the time, much harder. Determining what is demanded of us is the difficult part. Our vulnerability takes many forms, as does the vulnerability of those who care for us. Nothing can finally rid us of our fragile situation in the world. That we must experience alone. But it is caring, well and properly given, that can make it more endurable.

REFERENCES

Allmark, A. (1995). Can there be an ethics of care? *Journal of Medical Ethics* 21: 19–24.

Callahan, D. (1993). *The Troubled Dream of Life: In Search of a Peaceful Death.* New York: Simon & Schuster.

Cassell, E. (1991). *The Nature of Suffering and the Goals of Medicine.* New York: Oxford University Press.

Chin, A. E., Hedberg, K., Higginson, G. K., and Fleming, D. W. (1999). Legalized physician-assisted suicide in Oregon—the first year's experience. *New England Journal of Medicine* 340: 577–58.

Frank, A. (1991). *At the Will of the Body.* Boston: Houghton Mifflin.

Morse, J., Solberg, S., Neender, W., Bottorff, J., and Johnson, J. (1990). Concepts of caring and caring as a concept. *Advances in Nursing Science* 13(1): 1–14.

Selzer, R. (1995). "Imelda." In R. Reynolds and J. Stone, eds., *On Doctoring: Stories, Poems, Essays*, pp. 255–66. New York: Simon & Schuster.

Tolstoy, L. (1960). *The Death of Ivan Ilych and Other Stories.* New York: New American Library.

Veatch, R. (1998). The place of care in ethical theory. *Journal of Medicine and Philosophy* 23(2): 221–24.

2

Who Needs Caring?

A. E. BENJAMIN, PH.D.,
AND LEIGHTON E. CLUFF, M.D.

NEARLY ALL of us need caring and personal attention from others at certain times during our lives. Understanding, support, compassion, and comforting are particularly important to those individuals who have acute or chronic illnesses, or who are disabled and limited in their functional effectiveness. As we examine the various issues involved in caring, it is necessary to consider the range of individuals who need caring and the diversity of their situations.

This chapter begins with a brief overview of needs for caring among people who have acute health problems and illnesses. Then it examines the population groups with chronic illnesses and disabilities who are in need of persistent and long-term assistance, attention, support, and caring, as well as medical care—children, working-age adults with developmental disabilities, working-age adults with physical disabilities, persons with chronic mental illness, and frail older people. Although these groups have some common needs, we give separate attention to each group because variations among them can present different issues relevant to caring. We conclude by highlighting some of the factors that enable or tend to limit access to caring—family circumstances, social circumstances, the circumstances of modern health care, and economic circumstances.

ACUTE HEALTH PROBLEMS AND ILLNESSES

In addition to medical care, acute health problems and illnesses usually require caring from health professionals, family, and other members of the community. The sources and nature of caring, however, vary somewhat in accordance with particular types of acute problems and the stages in the life course at which they may arise.

All newborn babies, because of their vulnerability, have special needs for nurturing and bonding, whether in the hospital or at home. But low birth weight (LBW) newborns, who are at risk of medical problems, need caring especially. Overall, more than 7 percent of newborns have LBWs (2,500 grams or less). Almost 13 percent of births from teenage mothers are LBW infants, and among unmarried mothers the rate is 32.4 percent (*Statistical Abstract of the United States,* 1998). LBW babies most often are retained in an intensive care newborn nursery until it is certain that they will thrive at home with the mother. During this period of hospitalization, these infants require considerable attention and care from specially trained nurses, who play an important role in nurturing them, as well as in providing medical care. A mother who visits her baby in the intensive care unit may face considerable anxiety, especially if her child has a very low birth weight (VLBW). VLBW infants, who are at even greater risk of medical problems and disabilities, may be hospitalized for a long time and require intensive medical support in order to mature. Their mothers need continuing support, information, guidance, attention, and caring from their babies' physicians and nurses, even after taking the baby home.

Teenage and single mothers face additional problems, particularly when their children are ill or disabled, and require support from family and friends, as well as continuing support and assistance from health professionals. Vulnerable infants and children born to unmarried mothers have been a national concern for some years. In 1995, 13.1 percent of all births were to teenage mothers, more than half of them unmarried; 45 births per 1,000 were from unmarried women (*Statistical Abstract of the United States,* 1998). Support programs and groups have assisted these mothers, but such programs, alone, are often not enough. Without a spouse, the mother who is still in school or employed must depend on family members—especially a grandmother or great-grandmother—to assume much responsibility in caring, particularly when the baby is sick.

The most frequent acute illnesses experienced by children are infectious diseases (e.g., the common cold and influenza) and injuries. Most of the acute infections in children are relatively benign and rarely require medical care from a physician or nurse. They do, however, usually need attention and caring from parents, particularly mothers, who may find it necessary to be with the child continually to provide comfort and security. When the common infections of childhood and adolescence are severe, as may be the case for those who have asthma or serious chronic diseases such as cystic fibrosis or congenital abnormalities, most of their care will be in the home, even if a brief period of hospitalization is required. Parents play an essential role in ensuring that medication is taken as prescribed and that the child is comforted and cared for.

Injuries—such as fractures, sprains, open wounds and lacerations, and concussions—are perhaps the most important sources of acute health problems in infants, children, and teenagers. The rate of reported injuries for children under five years of age is 27 per 1,000, and the rate for those aged five to seventeen years is 30.2 per 1,000 (*Statistical Abstract of the United States,* 1998). Although the principal need of injured children may be medical care, they often require considerable assistance, attention, and support until fully recovered.

Child abuse is a major national problem that creates acute and chronic care needs. Of reported cases, 23 percent involve physical abuse and 12.3 percent involve sexual abuse. Abused children, particularly those who are victims of sexual abuse, can experience acute problems that may produce long-lasting harm as well. Emerging standards of care for sexually abused children recognize that patience, compassion, and support from health care providers and from family, relatives, and friends are essential (Hymel and Jenny, 1996).

The reported rate of rape in female children under age twelve is 84.9 per 100,000, and the rate in children age twelve and older is 43.5 per 1,000 (*Statistical Abstract of the United States,* 1998). The victims critically require a great deal of understanding, support, and comfort if they are to recover and lead normal lives; their families and guardians also need caring.

Substance abuse among young persons is a national tragedy and presents enormous challenges for health care providers, educators, society, and parents and guardians. The abuse of alcohol, hallucinogens, cocaine, heroin, and other drugs can alter the behavior of the abusers and have an impact on their schoolmates, other young persons, and their families. Moreover, abuse of these agents has resulted in injury and death of the abusers and others, often through accidents or violent acts. While diagnosis and treatment of those who abuse drugs and alcohol is essential, support groups can also be helpful in terminating and preventing recurrent abuse.

Many acute conditions that affect children are also experienced by adults; for example, injuries are as prevalent in those aged from forty-five to seventy-five as in children (*Statistical Abstract of the United States,* 1998). The same is true for poisoning, both accidental and that resulting from suicide attempts. Patients with injuries and poisoning serious enough to result in hospitalization are likely to be acutely disabled for some time;

they need assistance and support from others, in addition to physicians, both during the acute stage of their conditions and during convalescence.

From age fifteen to forty-four, acute psychoses are the second most prevalent condition resulting in hospitalization. The substantial challenges of caring for these patients with this condition, as well as those with other mental illnesses, are discussed in chapter 3.

Cerebrovascular accidents, or strokes, are also highly prevalent among adults, particularly after age sixty-five. Although stroke is a cause of chronic disability, its onset is usually acute. Immediately following the acute episode, affected persons can be frightened and need comfort, companionship, and support, usually by family members when at home. Caring is often necessary during a prolonged period of convalescence, perhaps with persistent disability. Those persons who recover from an acute episode may be fearful of recurrences, will benefit from encouragement to maintain their efforts at rehabilitation, and need ongoing support to live a "normal" life. Much the same is true for those who experience myocardial infarctions and other acute episodes of illness.

Suicide, although not considered a disease per se, is a phenomenon especially prevalent among very old people. Individuals aged seventy-five and older have almost twice the suicide rate of those who are younger (*Statistical Abstract of the United States,* 1998). Suicide presents problems for families, relatives, and friends, who can suffer loss, grief, guilt, and the stigma often associated with suicide. Survivors need to be with those who are compassionate and demonstrate care and concern while accepting personal grief (Smith et al., 1995). Moreover, caring, support, and appropriate medication for those who are depressed—aged or young—may abort or prevent suicide attempts.

PERSONS WITH CHRONIC ILLNESSES AND DISABILITIES

Although the need for caring can occur intermittently throughout the life course and in a variety of settings, caring is needed over extended periods of time (usually years) for persons of any age who have serious chronic illnesses and disabilities, because they require continuous support in carrying out functions that are essential to daily life. The proportion of chronically ill and disabled persons residing in institutions has declined steadily in the past three decades (Goldman et al., 1992). Today, most of them live at home with families or in community residential settings

(Feder, 1999). Their need for caring and support from a spouse, children, other family members, and friends becomes especially important. In the absence of or in combination with support from these sources, people may choose to or need to rely upon formal, paid services. Even with formal and informal assistance, however, there may be a lack of support and caring, and the consequences may be deleterious.

Numerous forces can affect the likelihood of experiencing chronic illness and disabilities and the needs for caring that are frequently associated with them. Although such illnesses and disabilities are immediate sources of personal anguish and impairment, we have begun to understand that certain population characteristics can also determine how those affected, and their caregivers, deal with their situations.

Men are more likely to experience certain disabling conditions, especially injuries, earlier in life; women, who live longer, are more likely to need assistance later in their lives (Hoffman and Rice, 1996; LaPlante and Miller, 1992). Moreover, women frequently outlive their husbands, have no spouse or companion, and have less personal, social, and financial support at a time in their lives when these can be crucial to having a degree of independence (Wallace, Abel, and Stefanowicz, 1996).

Race, ethnicity, and culture are related to needs for caring and how families respond to those needs, interacting in complex ways with social class factors (see Markides and Wallace, 1996; Williams, Lavizzo-Mourey, and Warren, 1994). Rates of disability vary according to race and ethnicity (Bradsher, 1996; Kennedy, LaPlante, and Kaye, 1997). Even within broad racial and ethnic groupings there are substantial differences; for example, among Asian Americans there are substantial differences in rates among Chinese Americans, Japanese Americans, Vietnamese Americans, and Cambodian Americans.

Cultural differences are also associated with tendencies to use organized professional services to obtain supportive assistance, although recent evidence on this is somewhat contradictory (Wallace, Abel, and Stefanowicz, 1996). Various studies have shown that older African Americans use nursing homes less and home-based services more than the elderly population in general and that minority populations generally rely more on informal, unpaid (usually family) help (Mui and Burnette, 1994). Patterns of differences for Latinos tend to mirror those of African Americans but are less pronounced (Wallace et al., 1998). Less is known empirically about how racial and ethnic differences are associated with the use of formal, paid disability-related services. Group differences in knowledge of available services, provider discrimination, and cultural expectations are among possible explanations for variations in the use of formal services and family support (Wallace, Abel, and Stefanowicz, 1996; Moon, Lubben, and Villa, 1998).

How Many Americans Are Chronically Ill and Disabled?

The extent of need for caring can probably be best understood in terms of the level of activity at which persons with chronic illnesses and disabilities can function in daily life. Estimates of the number of Americans who are dependent in their daily activities because of chronic illnesses and conditions vary widely, ranging from 99 million to 41 million (Hoffman and Rice, 1996; U.S. Bureau of the Census, 1997). The reasons for such discrepancies are that different sources of data use different definitions of disability and need, and the purposes for which the estimates are made vary widely (U.S. General Accounting Office, 1999). Although it is clear that many people in the United States report some type of chronic condition, fewer than half of them are limited in their daily lives by these conditions. Among those that are limited, fewer still are unable to carry out their *major* activities (e.g., going to school or work). In the mid-1990s, the population of persons limited in their major activity numbered between 24 million and 28 million (Bradsher, 1996; Hoffman and Rice, 1996; U.S. Bureau of the Census, 1997).

There seems to be limited consensus about what constitutes a *severe* disability (U.S. General Accounting Office, 1999). But various analysts estimate that between 12 and 13 million Americans of all ages are unable to carry out everyday activities without assistance from others, including about 2.4 million living in institutions (U.S. General Accounting Office, 1994). Other estimates suggest that about 7.3 million persons aged fifteen and over and living in the community have difficulty performing one or more activities of daily living—bathing, dressing, getting out of a chair or bed, toileting, or feeding oneself. Within this group, about half (3.7 million) require the assistance of another person to perform these core daily activities (Kennedy, LaPlante, and Kaye, 1997). In addition, needs for assistance stem from inability to perform instrumental activities of daily living such as managing finances, telephoning, shopping, preparing light meals, and being able to go outside the home independently. The most recent federal estimates of noninstitutionalized adults put the number of those with the most severe disability at 2.3 million (U.S. General Accounting Office, 1999). It is clear that the functionally disabled population that needs caring is large and growing, even as the debate continues regarding the precise size of the populations with the most severe needs (Binstock, Cluff, and von Mering, 1996).

The many different persons among the large number with long-term illnesses and disabilities have common and diverse caring needs. The variety of complex issues that arise for them and those who care for them are considered next, in some detail.

Common Needs

Although there are many diverse groups with severe disabilities, some of their commonalities are especially important to note in order to understand their needs for caring (Newcomer and Benjamin, 1997). For instance, people with severe disabilities are considerably less well off than the general population. Adults with disabilities are more likely than others to have less than a high school education and are far less likely to work (see figure 2.1). Only 26 percent of those aged twenty-one to sixty-four with severe disabilities have a job or business, compared with 82 percent of those with no disability (Stoddard et al., 1998). When those aged eighteen to twenty-one are included, the percentage of the severely disabled who are not unemployed or do not participate in the workforce drops to about 16 percent (U.S. General Accounting Office, 1994). As a consequence, adults with severe disabilities tend to have fewer material resources on which to draw as they manage their lives. Specifically, they are almost twice as likely as the general population to live in a household with an income of less than $20,000 (U.S. General Accounting Office, 1999). Limited resources and relative social isolation are more likely to be correlates of severe disability, whatever the source of that disability. These circumstances clearly influence the particular needs of disabled individuals and their dependency on caring families or available formal and organized services.

Disability is defined by limitations that hinder performance, entailing a loss of independence. Therein lies a paradox. Disabled persons require assistance with the most intimate aspects of daily life so that they can sustain and enhance their independence with respect to other aspects of living. Yet, according to various observers, such assistance can further dependence, rather than foster independence, depending on how it is organized and provided (Batavia, DeJong, and McKnew, 1991; Simon-Rusinowitz and Hofland, 1993). Whether disabling conditions are physical or mental, and whether among children, working age adults, or older persons, issues of

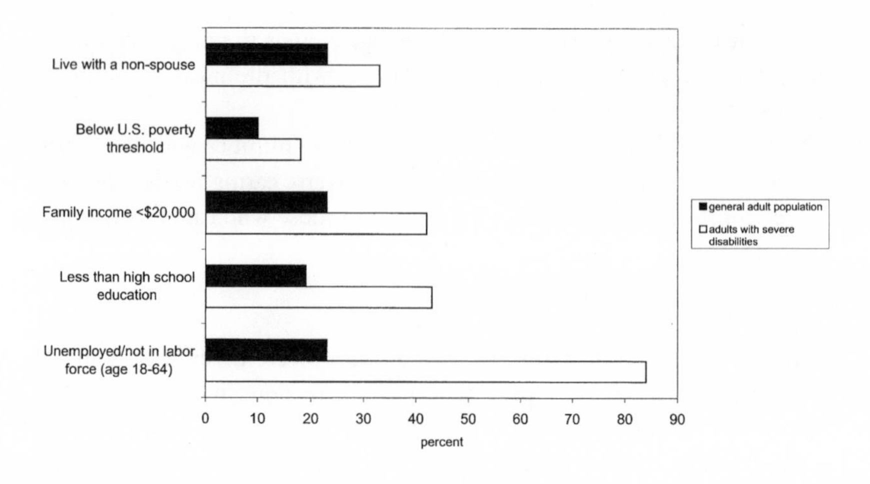

Figure 2.1. *Ratio of Adults with Severe Disabilities to the General Adult Population*

Source: National Health Interview Survey, 1994–95

choice and control permeate supportive caring services much more than medical services.

Diverse Needs

Commonalities among people with disabilities cannot mask the diversity and intensity of conditions, circumstances, and caring needs that characterize them. People acquire disabilities via myriad paths (see table 2.1), and a vast range of chronic physical and mental disorders, injuries, or impairments can limit capacity to perform essential daily activities (LaPlante, 1996). Moreover, the kinds of supportive assistance needed by children with special health needs, adults with chronic mental illness, and the frail elderly are not identical in type or intensity. This diversity and intensity is complicated because not all disabling conditions are stable; they fluctuate in the short term and over the long term. For example, a person with AIDS, multiple sclerosis, or rheumatoid arthritis may be functional during some days or weeks and impaired during others. The need for assistance and personal support may not be constant across time (although the need for monitoring may be).

People with disabilities also vary in terms of the types of activities for which assistance is needed. For example, as noted above, the need for as-

Table 2.1. *Most Common Conditions Causing Activity Limitation*

Rank	Conditions	Number (1,000s)	Percent of All Conditions
	All conditions	61,047	100.0
1	Heart disease	7,932	13.0
2	Deformities, orthopedic impairments, and disorders of the spine or back	7,672	12.6
3	Osteoarthrosis and allied disorders	5,048	8.3
4	Orthopedic impairment of lower extremity	2,817	4.6
5	Asthma	2,592	4.2
6	Diabetes	2,569	4.2
7	Mental disorders excluding learning disability and mental retardation	2,035	3.3
8	Disorders of the eye	1,577	2.6
9	Learning disability and mental retardation	1,575	2.6
10	Cancer	1,342	2.2
11	Visual impairments	1,294	2.1
12	Orthopedic impairment of shoulder and/or upper extremities	1,196	2.0
13	Other unknown and unspecified causes	1,188	1.9
14	Hearing impairments	1,175	1.9
15	Cerebrovascular disease	1,174	1.9

Source: National Center for Health Statistics, 1994.

sistance and caring can vary by age. Children are involved in play and school; most working-age adults want to be involved in employment; and most older people, while no longer working or raising children, seek to be active in various ways associated with retirement. The design of caring activities must take into account these differences.

Although some "laying on of hands"—as an expression of concern and understanding—is often essential to render caring, people with disabilities differ in the extent of their need for hands-on physical assistance, supervision and guidance for cognitive or psychological needs, and nursing and paramedical care for medical conditions that may involve supportive equipment and medications. Even though the boundaries between these areas of need are not precise, the dominance of one or another area can define the nature of caring and the patient's sense of independence. The presence of cognitive impairment can have a profound impact on the nature of caring and on the demands and rewards of caring relationships. The use of professional services, assistive equipment, and medications may provide more independence for the patient but can also bring about more dependence on caring persons who are required to administer or manage them.

As suggested earlier, most people with serious disabilities receive needed care from family members and friends; however, assistance from organized professional sources has been growing substantially over the past fifteen years (see Binstock and Cluff, 2000a). Whatever the source of professional assistance, the needs for caring associated with disability require a great deal of flexibility. For example, when medical monitoring is required, as well as supportive services, service planning is complex. For persons who must rely on organized professional services, flexible programming is a continuing challenge to public officials and health care administrators who are accountability-oriented and budget-sensitive.

Since generalizations such as these do not fully capture the diversity of disability or the challenges of caring and organized professional services, it is important to consider in more detail the needs of those population groups most in need. These include children with special health needs; adults with developmental disabilities; adults with physical disabilities; adults with chronic mental illness; and older persons with chronic conditions.

Children with Chronic Illness and Disabilities. Among children under age eighteen, about 8 percent of boys and 6 percent of girls have disabilities. About 2 percent of all children have severe functional limitations that require sustained, supportive caring from family and others (Kaye et al., 1996). Commonly referred to as "children with special health needs," this population has grown as medical technology has made survival possible for children who not long ago would have died at birth or in early childhood or adolescence (see Perrin, Shayne, and Bloom, 1993; Perrin, 1997). More than 90 percent of children with severe chronic conditions are estimated to survive into adulthood, and only a small percentage (perhaps 5%) does so with the assistance of major technologies.

Although most children with chronic physical disability do not have associated cognitive impairments, those with both conditions may require an extensive array of caring and supportive services at home and in educational and community settings. For example, physical and cognitive disabilities can interfere with school performance. In addition, psychiatric and behavioral problems are more common among children with chronic physical conditions (Perrin, 1997).

Children with special health needs thus may require caring not only from families but on other fronts as well—medical and nursing, mental health, educational, and social services. Typically, families provide substantial amounts of the care for children with disabilities, while also engaging in significant coordination of activities across organized service sectors (Perrin, Shayne, and Bloom, 1993; Benjamin, Matthias, and Franke, 1998). The intensity of supportive services needed typically ranges from continual monitoring to constant assistance and support.

Asthma, for example, is a chronic disease characterized by acute episodes with severe respiratory difficulty and airway obstruction. It is one of the more frequent conditions (4.2 per 100) responsible for hospitalization of children (*Statistical Abstract of the United States,* 1998). Medical management of childhood asthma is very important, but much of the care that is required is provided by parents and, sometimes, by teachers and school nurses. When the parent is well informed by a physician about the care needed at home, the child's asthma is more likely to be controlled and hospitalization avoided. Acute asthma attacks at home or at school can be frightening events. Calm and confidence exhibited by a parent, teacher, or other person is important in order to avoid having the child's asthma worsen because of fear and anxiety. In a way, the caring provided by a parent at home, with information provided by a caring physician, can go far in helping to keep an asthmatic child well.

Children with serious chronic diseases present considerable caring challenges for parents. The child may be hospitalized frequently and then returned home, where the parents, usually the mother, has the ongoing twenty-four-hour responsibility to meet the child's needs. This may require administration of medication or the use of technology such as an oxygen-supply system. Moreover, the parent must provide comfort, compassion, and support in order for the child to survive or thrive and mature. For some parents this presents a very difficult burden.

Caring parents feel isolated, uncertain about professional services and relationships, and anxious about the future of living circumstances and quality of care for their children (Krumholtz, 1993). In this situation, mothers and fathers need support and caring from each other as well as from their other children, relatives, friends, neighbors, religious congregations and clergy, and other community support groups. Programs such as Family Friends, directed by the National Council on the Aging, provide trained older volunteers to support and assist such parents, by caring for seriously disabled and chronically ill children in the home (National Council on the Aging, 1999). Family Friends has not only been useful in providing assistance in caring for a seriously ill or disabled child, but also has been most useful in supporting parents. Moreover, those who volunteer their services are benefited as well (Rinck, Naragon, and St. Clair, 1996).

Among infants and children, 313,000 under the age of five and 813,000 young persons between fifteen and twenty-one years of age have a serious developmental disability (*Statistical Abstract of the United States,* 1998). Most often, these disabilities are characterized by mental retardation, autism, and cerebral palsy. Those who are less severely disabled may be able to have an independent life and work. For the more severely disabled, however, parents and society must bear a long-lasting responsibility for providing them with support and assistance. For some, institutional care may be necessary because they do not have a home environment in which they can receive the caring they need. Parents or guardians of severely disabled children who remain at home face an extended period during which their lives are virtually committed to caring. Special schools and other programs may be available for the child, but at home parents must carry the burdens and (for some) the pleasures of caring.

Because developmentally disabled children and adolescents are often enrolled ("mainstreamed") in public schools along with "normal" students, teachers and administrators as well as school nurses have responsibilities to provide support and caring for them in this environment. Often, these educators are not prepared to meet the caring needs placed upon them and would benefit from guidance, instruction, and assistance in providing support. Meeting the caring needs of these children and adolescents must be done without compromising their education and the education of other students.

Adults with Developmental Disabilities. From 2 to 3 percent of the U.S. population is identified as having mental retardation or developmental disability during the pre-adult years, while a much smaller number (perhaps half of 1%) are considered to be moderately to profoundly retarded into adulthood. Relatively few adults in this category (i.e., with IQs of 50 or below) achieve full independence, although some may develop a range of self-care and employment skills.

Mental retardation is defined by the discrepancies between individual behavior and societal expectations about behavior appropriate to a given age. Those who are mentally retarded may require assistance and support in self-care, language, learning, mobility, self-direction, capacity for independent living, and economic self-sufficiency. Caring for this population involves not merely offering assistance and support but also providing opportunities to learn and practice culturally appropriate, and age-appropriate, behavior and skills (Lakin, 1997). Consequently, developmental disability involves cognitive support, training, and supervision, as well as assistance with physical needs. Family caregivers and institutional personnel caring for mentally impaired individuals have major caring responsibilities.

The majority of people with profound retardation live in residential institutions and nursing homes. But in the 1990s, the concept of "supported community living" introduced a significant shift in how care is designed and operationalized with this population. Supported community living emphasizes individual preferences and choices, providing people a home of their own, building on natural support systems, and providing formal services in personalized and nonintrusive ways. Although relatively few people with developmental disabilities currently participate in supported living (Lakin, 1997), the emphasis this model places on personal choice, community living, and independence have redefined and broadened care for this population to encompass caring. However, the involvement of family in caring for a retarded family member in these settings can be difficult.

Adults with Physical Disabilities. Developments in modern medicine and rehabilitation have greatly enhanced the chances that adults with physical disabilities caused by disease and injury will survive and, with needed support from family and others, lead productive lives. Many whose chances for survival were severely limited three to four decades ago are now likely to live into old age. The many specific impairments that underlie disabilities in persons aged eighteen to sixty-four vary by age, gender, and race and ethnicity (see Kemp, 1997; Such, Yelin, and Criswell, 1997; LaPlante, 1996).

Usually, chronic diseases are not static, and a majority of those with serious disabilities experience substantial changes over time in their illness and functional ability (Kemp, 1997). The dynamic nature of many disabilities presents a challenge to an organized service system that is more geared to treatment and rehabilitation at the onset of disability than to ongoing monitoring and systematic adaptation of services and assistive equipment to changing needs (Kemp, 1997). Under these circumstances, support, assistance, and caring by family members and friends may be especially important over the long haul.

Home-based personal-assistance services, assistive devices, adaptive housing, and assisted transportation are critically needed, but they are inaccessible for many people who can benefit from them (Kemp, 1997). The availability of these services varies widely across states and communities, even with the growth over time in federal funding for these benefits. Nonelderly adults who have not qualified for Medicare, as well as their caring families, must be concerned about sources of financing for both medical and supportive needs; the extent of their concern will depend on family income and other financial resources, whether they qualify for Medicaid, the generosity of their particular state Medicaid program, and many other factors. The absence of caring persons to support and assist under these circumstances can be devastating.

In part because the system of formally organized care is oriented to medical and rehabilitative treatment (rather than caring and support through social services), many adults under the age of sixty-five, like their elderly counterparts, rely on family members to meet their assistance needs and provide support following the onset of disability. In addition to the well-documented physical, psychological, and economic burdens of caring over long periods of time (Stone, Cafferata, and Sangl, 1987), families are facing new challenges in dealing with and planning for the aging of younger adults, increasing numbers of whom have survived illness and trauma and will outlive their family (especially parental) caregivers (Ansello, 1988; Kemp, 1997).

Adults with Chronic Mental Illness. An estimated 1 percent of the adult population experiences recurrent episodes of mental illness, most notably schizophrenia (Steinwachs, Kasper, and Lehman, 1997). While severe, acute episodes of mental illness can require immediate clinical attention, periods of persistent disability demand a range of coordinated responses from families, community service systems, and health care professionals. The duration, range, and severity of symptoms vary widely. But illnesses such as schizophrenia can be persistent in the absence of medical treatment. In order to control behavioral and destructive problems, clinical monitoring and medications are crucial elements of care. Indeed, pharmacotherapeutic strategies are central to assisting people with chronic mental conditions in managing their symptoms. The availability of these medications has made it feasible for more people to live at home and in the community and become functionally effective. This has mitigated the burden of caring that families face.

At the heart of strategies for community living are "social-skills training," supportive housing, and supportive employment. Social-skills training involves group treatment that targets the social disabilities that accompany chronic mental illness. Training emphasizes communications skills, assertiveness skills, problem-solving skills, and skills related to self-care. "Supported housing programs" emphasize mainstream housing integrated into the community with professional services provided as needed. Emphasis is placed on individual choice and normalization of the living environment. Supported employment programs for persons with chronic mental illness represent an alternative to traditional transitional and sheltered vocational rehabilitation programs. This model is intensive and highly individualized (Steinwachs, Kasper, and Lehman, 1997). These specialized approaches to caring for people with chronic mental illness, however, are not universally available. As a consequence, considerable responsibility falls on the family. (For a discussion of the burdens of family caring for persons with severe and persistent mental illness, see chapter 3.)

Older People with Chronic Needs. The prevalence of need for caring among adults with chronic conditions increases sharply with age, particularly at older ages. Although many older people are relatively healthy and functionally independent, persons aged sixty-five and older nonetheless represent about six of ten people with disabilities. Older persons experience dependence in basic activities of daily life at about twice the rate of those in the older working-age range (aged forty-five to sixty-four) and at four times the rate of the younger working-age group. Among those aged eighty-five and older, about 23 percent need personal assistance with at least one intimate activity of daily life such as dressing or toileting (Kennedy, LaPlante, and Kaye, 1997; Kassner and Bectel, 1998).

Most of the leading causes of functional impairment among older people are related to chronic illnesses (National Center for Health Statistics, 1993). An estimated 80 percent of persons aged sixty-five and older have at least one chronic disease, and for many the presence of two or more conditions complicates care planning. For some conditions, the benefit of medical treatment has been well confirmed (e.g., hypertension). For other conditions (e.g., stroke) functional outcomes can be improved with rehabilitation services. For still others (e.g., arthritis) assistive devices like canes and walkers may be useful in maintaining level of functioning, while caring and assistance from others may be necessary to maintain personal hygiene, dressing, eating, and preparing food (Such, Yelin, and Criswell, 1997).

When cognitive impairment due to dementing illness is present as a "co-morbid" condition, the complexity of caring can grow dramatically. Needs associated with dementia are personal and social, as well as medical. At the least, affected persons are likely to need supervision of their daily activities, and as cognitive impairment increases, the range of needs is likely to include not only full-time supervision but also assistance with basic activities like eating (Luxenberg and Newcomer, 1997). (For a fuller discussion of the care needs of older adults who are chronically ill and disabled, as well as a consideration of issues of caring involved with this population, see chapters 3, 7, and 8.)

FACTORS AFFECTING ACCESS TO CARING

Before concluding this discussion of "who needs caring?" it is important to consider the factors that affect access—for the acutely ill, and the chronically ill and disabled—to the compassion, understanding, and support that caring comprises. Among these factors are family circumstances, the social environment in which one lives, the forces that shape the nature of modern health care, special issues affecting disabled people who rely on paid services for personal assistance, and the economic circumstances of individuals and the collective mechanisms that can finance supportive caring.

Family Circumstances

The family remains the most prominent resource available to most people who need caring. This seems to be true, generally, in terms of illness and disability, across age groups, and in the amount and quality of care. However, the extent to which families are able (and willing) to provide caring does vary in relation to various groups that need supportive care.

It is no surprise that parents are the primary sources of care for children. Not only do most parents want to assume this role, but societal expectations place pressures on the family to provide and manage caring, both through common norms about parental responsibility and through the relative absence of financial resources to underwrite alternatives (Perrin, Shayne, and Bloom, 1993).

Working-age adults with physical disabilities, developmental disabilities, or chronic mental health problems are in more uncertain territory with respect to family care. Most adults with disabilities want to be independent, productive, and self-sufficient. But over time, many have become dependent upon family resources to supplement what are frequently inadequate public benefits, including income assistance, medical assistance, housing, and transportation. On average, dependence on family care may be lowest among those with physical disabilities and highest among those with severe mental illness.

Older people with physical and/or cognitive and mental disabilities usually depend on caring family members, especially spouses and children. But societal expectations concerning family obligations toward the elderly are mixed. While society values a familial commitment to care, adult children who might undertake caring are also encouraged to pursue job opportunities, raise and nurture children, and plan for their future relatively free of obligations to an earlier generation. These competing commitments, along with the extent of family financial resources and the physical and psychological capacity to care for others, will change over time, and not necessarily in ways that are consonant with the changing needs of older people with disabilities.

Single Parents. In 1998, there were more than 6 million female-headed households and more than 1 million male-headed households responsible for children under age eighteen, but with no spouse present (*Statistical Abstract of the United States,* 1998). Among parents who had no spouse, persons fifteen to twenty-four years of age were responsible for 2.5 million children.

Caring for children can be difficult when a single parent is employed. When a child is acutely ill, for example, the parent is faced with the dilemma of either leaving work to care for the child or remaining at work. In the latter case, either the child is neglected or the working mother or father must depend on others (and often be unsure about the quality of caring that the child receives). This dilemma spread to more single parent families during the 1990s as national and state efforts to reduce welfare rolls led greater numbers of poor single parents to become employed. Fortunately, some private-sector employers, states, and the federal government have provided resources and established programs that enable children of these parents to receive care (see chapter 11).

Relatives of the mother or father, other mothers, friends and neighbors, and child care centers can provide assistance, but they may or may not be effective in caring. Foster care of children provided by relatives has expanded in past decades. Almost 3 million children are the responsibility of grandparents (*Statistical Abstract of the United States,* 1998). But, foster care for preterm and other infants of single parents places them at risk. They often receive inadequate health care, having fewer acute care visits to physicians, and are more frequently rehospitalized (Gennaro, York, and Dunphy, 1998).

Moving to a New Locale. In recent years, the geographical mobility of many, including women in childbearing years, has increased (*Statistical Abstract of the United States,* 1998), often resulting in separation of parent(s) and children from grandparents, other relatives, and friends. A move to a distant locale can make it exceedingly difficult, for a time, to identify persons who could and will provide support and caring for the children.

Leaving the Family. As children mature into young adults they leave home and often lack the immediate supportive environment of families and friends. For young persons with severe disabilities, this can be a particularly stressful transition, especially when they go away to colleges and universities. The physical environments of these educational institutions have been increasingly modified in recent decades in order to provide facile movement about campus for physically disabled students. But the support, compassionate treatment, and concern they may require can be lacking, both from the educational institutions required under law (the Americans with Disabilities Act) to provide supportive services and from their fellow students. Able-bodied students may find it difficult to associate with seriously disabled students who are unable to participate in physical activities such as dancing and athletics and who may not appear to be suitable companions to the opposite sex. On the other hand, it is impressive how many students on a college or university campus are sensitive to the supportive and compassionate needs of disabled students and provide some measure of caring for them. For those students who become involved with seriously disabled classmates, the experience can be important to their subsequent, lifelong understanding and support for persons with disabilities.

The Family and Caring for Older Persons. Older persons who have never married, of course, have no spouse and may have no children available to undertake caring. Among married couples, older women, particularly those aged seventy-five and older, are less likely than older men to have a caring spouse. For every nine women in this age range there are about five men (Hobbs, 1996). In general, older women are more likely to be living alone and too poor to afford paid services for their care needs (*Statistical Abstract of the United States,* 1998).

Today's extended life expectancy has resulted in increasing numbers of four-generation families (Bengtson, Rosenthal, and Burton, 1990). It is becoming common for very old and impaired parents to look for caring and support from their elderly children. However, when elderly children are impaired themselves, the challenges of caring for one or two parents may be too much for them. In such cases, children in the third generation of the family may find the problems of caring both for parents and grandparents overwhelming.

Younger adult children also confront substantial difficulties in being able to provide caring for a parent at the level to which they aspire. Middle-aged women, in particular, often confront the multiple challenges of maintaining their jobs, caring for their children (and in some circumstances, an ill spouse), and caring for their parents and parents-in-law (Brody, 1990). In addition, substantial geographical distance from parents can sharply inhibit the caring capacities of children.

Various living arrangements can compensate for and complement family circumstances that are not optimal for caring for disabled older persons. Assisted-living facilities and continuing-care retirement communities can provide some measure of personal support (see chapter 8). And nursing homes are available for those who cannot be maintained in the home because of their functional limitations (see chapter 7). Similarly, paid home care services and programs such as Meals on Wheels, senior citizen centers, and adult day care centers can meet many of the specific needs of impaired older persons.

Social Circumstances

Even when family members and neighbors are nearby, one can be "alone." Not all families and neighbors are willing or prepared to provide the support, understanding, and compassion that people with care needs may require. The affected person may be as isolated and alone at home with family or friends nearby as they might be if family and friends were far away. Under these circumstances, some aged persons and children may be neglected and even abused. Much the same can be said of battered women (Rodriquez et al., 1996).

Religious and other volunteer organizations can provide some of the support and caring needed for those who are, in effect, alone (see chapter 9); for example, religious congregations and clergy minister to the support of and caring for those in the community who are in need (Cluff and Cluff, 1983). Faith in Action, a program funded by the Robert Wood Johnson Foundation, assists religious congregations in developing such programs. Presently, more than a thousand of these programs throughout the country seek to meet personal care needs and provide compassionate care and support for frail and disabled persons who reside in their own homes (Jellinek, Appel, and Keenan, 1999).

Sick and disabled persons who are alone or isolated from friends and family in large "inner cities" can have a very difficult time when in need of support and caring. In recent years there has been a substantial growth in the number of inner-city men and women who are poor, substance abusers, or have AIDS (Osborne, 1992). Although such persons—dwelling in single-room-occupancy establishments, or homeless—live in the midst of their fellow human beings, in areas where medical facilities are available and many social-service programs operate, society too often seems to ignore their presence and their needs. For a variety of reasons, families may not feel responsible for members who are in desperate need; or, if they feel responsible, their own life circumstances may preclude their being as supportive and caring as they might like to be. Even neighbors in adjacent rooms or apartments in inner cities may neglect the presence of one nearby who is in need of support and compassion. (Religious and secular holidays can be particularly difficult times.)

Although society has reportedly been experiencing "compassion fatigue" regarding the plight of the homeless and other isolated inner-city vulnerable persons, apparently the public has not lost compassion for them (Link et al., 1995). Volunteer groups, especially religious groups, contribute much to help meet the needs of these populations. Programs have been established in a number of communities, providing shelter, caring, and support for the homeless and substance abusers (see, e.g., Robert Wood Johnson Foundation, 1999). These efforts represent important contributions of society in providing support and compassionate understanding for those who are alone and in need.

The ill and disabled in small-town or rural settings may be the recipients of caring from sources other than family more than those who live in the inner city. In rural areas, people typically know each other, work together, go to the same church, and are familiar with each others' successes, failures, and problems. In many such communities (though not always) people tend to look out for one another (see chapter 9).

When a rural resident cannot manage to get to the nearest physician, perhaps located in another town, members of the community will often assist with transportation. The same is true when access to a distant hospital is needed. However, in rural areas hospitals are often far removed geographically from family and friends. In such circumstances, support and compassion from hospital staff are especially needed.

The Circumstances of Modern Health Care

Enormous advances in medical science and technology have improved medicine's ability to alleviate and cure disease, both acute and chronic. But listening, compassion, and support for the patient and family have almost become a thing of the past in physicians' offices, clinics, and hospitals.

Changes in the financing, organization, and delivery of medical care, and the modern armamentarium of diagnostic and therapeutic technologies, have had major effects on the opportunity and time available for physicians to provide the support, compassion, and understanding that most patients need and would like to receive (see chapters 5 and 6). Many physicians want to provide compassionate care for their patients, but the exigencies of medical practice today often make this impossible. Nurses, social workers, and other health care professionals—who work in physicians' offices, clinics, hospitals, nursing homes, and a variety of home- and community-based settings—are somewhat more able to provide the support that patients need. But their efforts to do so are often compromised by the same array of health system factors that affect physicians.

In the arena of long-term care, the economics and labor-force problems of most nursing homes are such that compassionate support and caring is often difficult to provide for residents (see chapter 7). Although professional home care services provide opportunities for nurses, therapists, and home health aides to know, support, and care for their patients, these services are financed, organized, and administered in fashions that limit these opportunities (Binstock and Cluff, 2000a).

Pharmacies are often a source of assistance to patients in situations (sometimes emergencies) requiring guidance, understanding support, and compassion. Today, the pharmacist is often accessible and available at times when other health care professionals are not. Moreover, pharmacists tend to be sympathetic when dealing with those who are ill and have health problems; they may seem to be less threatening or domineering than physicians (Casaurang, 1998).

Perhaps the one bastion that is fully committed to providing compassion, understanding, and caring is hospice programs, where the needs of dying persons are met (Moore and McCollough, 2000; Saunders and Kastenbaum, 1997). It is regrettable that such commitment is not realized in all the arenas of contemporary health care.

Caring by Professionals and Agencies: Special Issues for Disabled Persons

In any given year, the vast majority of people in the United States have some contact with the medical care system. Whether it is a routine examination, some tests, or minor surgery, medical interaction is a risky business, and most of us have experienced the sense of dependency and uncertainty associated with the patient role. For persons with disabilities, not only is the sense of vulnerability experienced in medical encounters amplified, but it also extends to other helping relationships and, indeed, to all aspects of living in which they seek to feel secure, enhance their autonomy, and gain a sense of personal fulfillment.

For those disabled persons who must rely on paid services from professionals and paraprofessionals (often involving service agencies) for personal assistance, caring raises some special issues. Most conceptions of caring focus on the family and health professionals, appropriately raising issues about the limitations of professional training that emphasizes the technical aspects of treatment at the expense of the human ones. To be sure, an emphasis on acute, post-acute, and rehabilitation services is highly relevant for people with disabilities, whose survival may depend upon these resources and who on average tend to be heavy users of medical care (Rice and LaPlante, 1992; Burns et al., 1990). However, when conceptions of professional health care are extended to supportive care, new issues emerge.

Public programs such as Medicare and Medicaid typically consider services like personal assistance to be an extension of medical care and thus available only with medical authorization and nursing supervision. This medical conception emphasizes the importance of professional design and management of services and standards of quality framed by professional norms. But this is only one conception of supportive care for people with disabilities.

Another model of supportive care emphasizes consumer direction and independent living, most notably in the context of personal-assistance services (for a fuller discussion of this model, see chapter 8). From this perspective, professionals should play no active role apart from determination of eligibility; instead, the disabled person should assume responsibility for recruiting, managing, and directing the caregiver. The disabled person is here considered a "consumer" rather than a "patient," in order to emphasize active decision making rather than the passive receipt of services. The caregiver in turn is considered to be an employee of the consumer and takes direction about how and when services are to be provided. This model places little emphasis on worker training. Since tasks like bathing and dressing are personal and have relatively minor technical components, consumer preferences are considered a sufficient basis for worker direction, and the worker can be accountable only to the consumer. The model also assumes that where cognitive impairment is involved, consumer capacity for full self-direction is limited but not necessarily eliminated, and a guardian or surrogate may help manage the personal-assistance relationship (Batavia, DeJong, and McKnew, 1991; Doty, Kasper, and Litvak, 1996).

Historically, younger adults with physical disabilities have been most vocal in calling for an emphasis on caring designed to foster independence and for a more prominent role for the client/consumer in the caring relationship. This perspective has also begun to influence thinking among those who design services for people with developmental disabilities and frail older people, and it has some important implications for how we think about the context of caring.

Analysts have given thoughtful attention to the nature of the helping relationship, elaborating the importance of empathy, sensitivity, and other virtues of the caregivers. They have also reminded us that caring should have a "goals" component, since care activity should be defined by the needs and aspirations of the person receiving care, rather than those of the caregiver alone. It is precisely on this point that advocates for consumer direction have taken Daniel Callahan's notion of the "particularity of caring" (see chapter 1) and made it the centerpiece of the caring relationship. They argue that the debate about appropriate professional roles for caregivers should shift to a more productive discussion about how to train people with disabilities to take charge of their own lives. They also argue that a hierarchical medical model with the physician-professional at the top should be replaced by a humanitarian-social model with the disabled consumer being in charge. Rather than struggle professionally over the place of individual patient goals ("particularity"), in the humanitarian-social model we are encouraged to transfer authority to consumers who can define their own preferences and make their own choices.

Ironically, in the context of an ascendant consumer-direction model, if the "helping professions" assume stronger nonmedical caring roles, their efforts in caring may come to emphasize client independence and self-determination. In this scenario, as professionals embrace the diverse goals of a caring relationship, attention would shift to the aspirations and preferences of the recipient and how to assist in achieving these. Conceptions would shift, from people with caring needs being *patients* to them being *consumers* and *decision makers* who make their own choices about how they live and die. This service scenario is not merely an abstraction: it has been tested and applied widely with diverse disabled populations, most often in the context of care at home (Benjamin, Matthias, and Franke, 2000; Cameron and Firman, 1995; Doty, Kasper, and Litvak, 1996).

Economic Circumstances

Finally, economic circumstances—both individual and collective—can limit access to caring. At the threshold, more than 44 million Americans do not have health insurance (U.S. Bureau of the Census, 1999). If they do seek health care, and are unable to pay for it, an emergency room will probably be where they receive it. In this setting, health care professionals are rushed and have little time for compassion, even if they are disposed to express it. Moreover, those who use emergency rooms for their care are not able to establish an ongoing, continuous relationship with a physician, which inhibits an essential ingredient of caring—some knowledge of the patient as a total person.

Many poor persons are eligible for Medicaid. But about half of them receive their health care in the context of managed care organizations (Fox, McManus, and Almeida, 1998), settings in which it is difficult to establish an ongoing patient/physician relationship (Emanuel and Dubler, 1995). In addition, poverty, near-poverty, and lower-income status limit the ability of families to provide caring. As discussed earlier in this chapter, responsibilities for caring compete with responsibilities to work and thereby maintain the family financially. Obtaining professional services to fill the gaps in family caring is financially impossible for such families (although some states have adopted the Medicaid personal-assistance benefit or have received special waivers from the federal government to provide supportive in-home services through the Medicaid program; see Doty, Kasper, and Litvak, 1996; Kane, Kane, and Ladd, 1998). Poverty can also, of course, have deleterious effects on the family's physical residence, neighborhood environment, and the quality of family life.

Even in many middle-class families, economic factors limit the quantity and quality of caring that they can provide. Employment obligations often make direct caring by family members difficult or impossible. Many employers do grant leaves-of-absence, lasting several months for new mothers and for more limited periods for employees with relatively short-term caring responsibilities. However, middle-class family members who have long-term caring responsibilities must rely on hiring personnel to fill the gaps; they frequently find that the cost of such support is formidable (Binstock and Cluff, 2000b).

The economics of America's health care system also tend to limit caring. The contemporary emphasis on economic accountability—in both the free market and public sectors—generates pressures that reduce opportunities for caring. As noted above, the financing and organization of health care leaves physicians and other health care professionals with little time and latitude for undertaking the levels of compassion, understanding, and support that most of them would like to provide for their patients.

The governments of a number of industrialized nations provide home care services as a universal entitlement (regardless of a family's financial means) and some also provide direct financial support to patients and their families in order to facilitate caring in the home, particularly for those who need long-term care (Kane, Kane, and Ladd, 1998; Monk and Cox, 1991). In the United States, however, there are no universal programs, and financial assistance is largely unavailable. A number of congressional bills have been introduced over the past dozen years to create a role for the federal government in this area. But they have not been enacted, largely because of the budgetary concerns that have dominated national politics in this period.

Among the nations of the world, the United States spends more of its gross domestic product on health care than any other nation (Anderson and Poullier, 1999). Most of this expenditure helps to create corporate and individual wealth; relatively little of it is devoted to the promotion of caring (see Leadership, 1998). In the twenty-first century, a major challenge for U.S. society will be to restructure its health care system so that we can become more of a caring society.

REFERENCES

Anderson, G. F., and Poullier, J.-P. (1999). Health spending, access, and outcomes: Trends in industrialized countries. *Health Affairs* 18(3): 178–92.

Ansello, E. F. (1988). The intersecting of aging and disabilities. *Educational Gerontology* 14: 351–64.

Batavia, A. I., DeJong, G., and McKnew, L. B. (1991). Toward a national personal assistance program: The independent living model of long-term care for persons with disabilities. *Journal of Health Politics, Policy, and Law* 16: 523–45.

Bengtson, V., Rosenthal, C., and Burton, L. (1990). Families and aging: Diversity and heterogeneity. In R. H. Binstock and L. K. George, eds., *Handbook of Aging and the Social Sciences,* 3rd ed., pp. 263–87. San Diego: Academic Press.

Benjamin, A. E., Matthias, R. E., and Franke, T. M. (1998). *Comparing Client-Directed and Agency Models for Providing Supportive Services at Home.* Report to the assistant secretary for planning and evaluation, U.S. Department of Health and Human Services. Los Angeles: School of Public Policy and Social Research, University of California, Los Angeles.

Benjamin, A. E., Matthias, R. E., and Franke, T. M. (2000). Comparing consumer-directed and agency models for providing supportive services at home. *Health Services Research* 35: 351–66.

Binstock, R. H., and Cluff, L. E., eds. (2000a). *Home Care Advances: Research and Policy Issues.* New York: Springer Publishing.

Binstock, R. H., and Cluff, L. E. (2000b). Issues and challenges in home care. In R. H. Binstock and L. E. Cluff, eds., *Home Care Advances: Research and Policy Issues,* pp. 3–34. New York: Springer Publishing.

Binstock, R. H., Cluff, L. E., and von Mering, O. (1996). Issues affecting the future of long-term care. In R. H. Binstock, L. E. Cluff, and O. von Mering, eds., *The Future of Long-Term Care: Social and Policy Issues,* pp. 3–18. Baltimore: Johns Hopkins University Press.

Bradsher, J. E. (1996). Disability among racial and ethnic groups. *Disability Statistics Abstract* #10. Washington, DC: National Institute of Disability and Rehabilitation Research (NIDRR).

Brody, E. M. (1990). *Women in the Middle: Their Parent-Care Years.* New York: Springer Publishing.

Burns, T. J., Batavia, A. I., Smith, Q. W., and DeJong, G. (1990). Primary health care needs of persons with physical disabilities. *Archives of Physical and Medical Rehabilitation* 71: 138–43.

Cameron, K., and Firman, J. (1995). *International and Domestic Programs Using "Cash and Counseling" Strategies to Pay for Long-Term Care.* Washington, DC: National Council on the Aging.

Casaurang, P. (1998). Multiple demands for assistance from pharmacists (Pharmacien, Le Kremlin-Bitetre). *Annales Pharmaceutiques Françaises* 56(4): 187–90.

Cluff, C. B., and Cluff, L. E. (1983). Informal support for disabled persons by religious and community organizations. *Journal of Chronic Disability* 36: 815–20.

Doty, P., Kasper, J., and Litvak, S. (1996). Consumer-directed models of personal care: Lessons from Medicaid. *Milbank Quarterly* 74: 377–409.

Emanuel, E. J., and Dubler, N. N. (1995). Preserving the physician-patient relationship in the era of managed care. *Journal of the American Medical Association* 273: 323–29.

Feder, J. (1999). The policy context for the long-term care debate. Paper presented at Princeton University, April 30, Conference on financing long-term care: Policy options and their economic impact, sponsored by the Council on the Economic Impact of Health System Change, Brandeis University, Waltham, MA.

Fox, H. B., McManus, M. A., and Almeida, R. A. (1998). Managed care's impact on Medicaid financing for early intervention services. *Health Care Financing Review* 20(1): 59–72.

Gennaro, S., York, R., and Dunphy, P. (1998). Vulnerable infants: Kinship care and health. *Pediatric Nursing* 24(2): 19–25.

Goldman, H. H., Morrissey, J. P., Ridgely, M. S., Frank, R. G., Newman, S. J., and Kennedy, C. (1992). Lessons from the program on chronic mental illness. *Health Affairs* 11(3): 51–68.

Hobbs, F. B. (1996). *65+ in the United States.* U.S. Bureau of the Census, Current Population Reports, Special Studies, P23-190. Washington, DC: U.S. Government Printing Office.

Hoffman, C., and Rice, D. P. (1996). *Chronic Care in America: A 21st Century Challenge.* Princeton, NJ: Robert Wood Johnson Foundation.

Hymel, K. P., and Jenny, C. (1996). Child sexual abuse. *Pediatrics in Review* 17(7): 236–49.

Jellinek, P., Appel, T. G., and Keenan, T. (1999). Faith in action: To improve health and health care, 1998–99. In S. L. Isaacs and J. R. Knickman, eds., *The Robert Wood Johnson Foundation Anthology*, pp. 111–41. Princeton, NJ: Robert Wood Johnson Foundation.

Kane, R. A., Kane, R. L., and Ladd, R. C. (1998). *The Heart of Long-Term Care.* New York: Oxford University Press.

Kassner, E., and Bectel, R. W. (1998). *Midlife and Older Americans with Disabilities: Who Gets Help? A Chartbook.* Washington, DC: Public Policy Institute, AARP.

Kaye, H. S., LaPlante, M. P., Carlson, D., and Wenger, B. L. (1996). Trends in disability rates in the United States, 1970–1994. *Disability Statistics Abstract* #17. Washington, DC: NIDRR.

Kemp, B. J. 1997. Care for adults with a disability, now and as they age. In R. J. Newcomer and A. E. Benjamin, eds., *Indicators of Chronic Health Conditions*, pp. 136–68. Baltimore: Johns Hopkins University Press.

Kennedy, J., LaPlante, M. P., and Kaye, H. S. (1997). Need for assistance in the activities of daily living. *Disability Statistics Abstract* #18. Washington, DC: NIDRR.

Krumholtz, H. A. (1993). Parents caring for young adults with severe physical disabilities. *Developmental Medicine and Child Neurology* 35(1): 24–32.

Lakin, K. C. (1997). Persons with developmental disabilities: Mental retardation as an exemplar. In R. J. Newcomer and A. E. Benjamin, eds., *Indicators of Chronic Health Conditions*, pp. 99–135. Baltimore: Johns Hopkins University Press.

LaPlante, M. P. (1996). Health conditions and impairments causing disability. *Disability Statistics Abstract* #16. Washington, DC: NIDRR.

LaPlante, M. P., and Miller, K. S. (1992). People with disabilities in basic life activities in the U.S. *Disability Statistics Abstract* #3. Washington, DC: NIDRR.

Leadership for a Healthy 21st Century, Health Care Forum (1998–99). *Health Forum Journal* supplement 1: 1–27.

Link, B. G., Schwartz, S., Moore, R., Phelan, J., Struening, E., Stueve, A., and Colten, M. E. (1995). Public knowledge, attitudes, and beliefs about homeless people: Evidence for compassion fatigue. *American Journal of Community Psychology* 23: 522–55.

Luxenberg, J. S., and Newcomer, R. J. (1997). Chronic illness among elderly people. In R. J. Newcomer and A. E. Benjamin, eds., *Indicators of Chronic Health Conditions*, pp. 201–34. Baltimore: Johns Hopkins University Press.

Manji, I. (1994). Meeting the needs of special-needs patients. *Journal of the Canadian Dental Association* 60: 489–90.

Markides, K. S., and Wallace, S. P. (1996). Health and long-term care needs of ethnic minority elders. In J. C. Romeis, R. M. Coe, and J. E. Morley, eds., *Applying Health Services Research to Long-Term Care*, pp. 23–42. New York: Springer Publishing.

Monk, A., and Cox, C. (1991) *Home Care for the Elderly: An International Perspective.* New York: Auburn House.

Moon, A., Lubben, J. E., and Villa, V. (1998). Awareness and utilization of community long-term services by elderly Korean and non-Hispanic White Americans. *Gerontologist* 38: 309–16.

Moore, C., and McCollough, R. H. (2000). Hospice: End-of-life care at home. In R. H. Binstock and L. E. Cluff, eds., *Home Care Advances: Research and Policy Issues,* pp. 101–16. New York: Springer Publishing.

Mui, A. C., and Burnette, D. (1994). Long-term care services used by frail elders: Is ethnicity a factor? *Gerontologist* 34: 190–98.

National Center for Health Statistics (1993). *Vital Health Statistics of the United States, 1991* supplement 42. Hyattsville, MD: U.S. Public Health Service.

National Center for Health Statistics (1994). *Current Estimates from the National Health Interview Survey, 1992.* Vital and Health Statistics, series 10, no. 189. Hyattsville, MD: U.S. Public Health Service.

National Council on the Aging (1999). Family Friends Project (accessed August 10, 1999).

Newcomer, R. J., and Benjamin, A. E. (1997). Community-level indicators for chronic health care services. In R. J. Newcomer and A. E. Benjamin, eds., *Indicators of Chronic Health Conditions,* pp. 302–45. Baltimore: Johns Hopkins University Press.

Northam, E. A. (1997). Chronic illness in children. *Journal of Pediatric Child Health* 33: 369–72.

Osborne, J. E. (1992). AIDS and the politics of compassion, National Commission on AIDS. *Hospitals* 66(18): 64.

Perrin, J. M. (1997). Children with chronic health conditions. In R. J. Newcomer and A. E. Benjamin, eds., *Indicators of Chronic Health Conditions,* pp. 69–98. Baltimore: Johns Hopkins University Press.

Perrin, J. M., Shayne, M. W., and Bloom, S. R. (1993). *Home and Community Care for Chronically Ill Children.* New York: Oxford University Press.

Rice, D. P., and LaPlante, M. P. (1992). Medical expenditures for disability and disabling comorbidity. *American Journal of Public Health* 82: 739–41.

Rinck, C., Naragon, P., and St. Clair, J. (1996). *Family Friends: A National Evaluation of Six Administration on Aging Sites.* Kansas City: University of Missouri–Kansas City, Institute for Human Development.

Robert Wood Johnson Foundation (1999). The healing place. *Advances* (Jan. 29): 3.

Rodriquez, M. A., Quiroga, S. S., and Bauer, H. M. (1996). *Archives of Family Medicine* 5(3): 153–58.

Saunders, C., and Kastenbaum, R. (1997). *Hospice Care on the International Scene.* New York: Springer Publishing.

Simon-Rusinowitz, L., and Hofland, B. F. (1993). Adopting a disability approach to home care services for older adults. *Gerontologist* 33: 159–67.

Smith, B. J., Mitchell, A. M., Bruno, A. A., and Constantino, R. E. (1995). Exploring widows' experiences after the suicide of their spouse. *Journal of Psychosocial Nursing and Mental Health Services* 33(5): 10–15.

Statistical Abstract of the United States. (1998). 118th ed. Washington, DC: U.S. Bureau of the Census.

Steinwachs, D. M., Kasper, J., and Lehman, A. (1997). Care for individuals with severe mental illness. In R. J. Newcomer and A. E. Benjamin, eds., *Indicators of Chronic Health Conditions,* pp. 235–59. Baltimore: Johns Hopkins University Press.

Stoddard, S., Jans, L., Ripple, J. M., and Kraus, L. (1998). *Chartbook on Work and Disability in the United States, 1998.* An InfoUse Report. Washington, DC: NIDRR.

Stone, R. I., Cafferata, G. L., and Sangl, J. (1987). Caregivers of the frail elderly: A national profile. *Gerontologist* 27: 616–26.

Such, C. L., Yelin, E. H., and Criswell, L. A. (1997). Adults with chronic disease:

Musculoskeletal conditions as an exemplar. In R. J. Newcomer and A. E. Benjamin, eds., *Indicators of Chronic Health Conditions*, pp. 169–200. Baltimore: Johns Hopkins University Press.

U.S. Bureau of the Census (1997). *One in Ten Americans Reported a Severe Disability in 1994–95*. Census Bureau Reports, CB97-148. Washington, DC: U.S. Department of Commerce.

U.S. Bureau of the Census (1999). *Health Insurance Coverage: 1998*. Current Population Reports: Consumer Income, P60-208. Washington, DC: U.S. Government Printing Office.

U.S. General Accounting Office (1994). *Long-Term Care: Diverse, Growing Population Includes Millions of Americans of All Ages* (GAO/HEHS-95-26). Washington, DC: U.S. Government Printing Office.

U.S. General Accounting Office (1999). *Adults with Severe Disabilities: Federal and State Approaches for Personal Care and Other Services* (GAO/HEHS-99-101). Washington, DC: U.S. Government Printing Office.

Wallace, S. P., Abel, E. K., and Stefanowicz, P. (1996). Long term care and the elderly. In R. M. Andersen, T. H. Rice, and G. F. Kominski, eds., *Changing the U.S. Health Care System: Key Issues in Health Services, Policy, and Management*, pp. 180–201. San Francisco: Jossey-Bass.

Wallace, S. P., Levy-Storms, L., Kington, R. S., and Andersen, R. M. (1998). The persistence of race and ethnicity in the use of long-term care. *Journal of Gerontology* 53B: S104–12.

Williams, D. R., Lavizzo-Mourey, R., and Warren, R. C. (1994). The concept of race and health status in America. *Public Health Reports* 109: 26–41.

3

Caring and Mental Illness

BURTON V. REIFLER, M.D., M.P.H.,
AND NANCY J. COX, M.S.W.

In one of the most famous essays in medicine, Francis Peabody spoke eloquently about the human side of patient care, and made his often-quoted statement, "One of the essential qualities of the clinician is interest in humanity, for the secret of the care of the patient is in caring for the patient" (Peabody, 1927: 882). Interestingly, buried in the essay, "The Care of the Patient," is a mild criticism of caring as provided by families, where he echoes sentiments widely held at that time by referring to the patient as "a gentle invalid overawed by a dominating family." Now, three-quarters of a century later, we have learned that Peabody's statement needs modification. In fact, the secret of caring for the patient, particularly individuals with mental illness, lies in caring for both the patient and the caregiver.

Caring for people with mental illness carries the same demands, expectations, and rewards as caring for those with physical illness. It involves assistance in daily activities of living and, ideally, compassion, sympathy, concern, feeling, and emotional support. But misunderstandings about mental illness throughout our society create special burdens and problems that make caring for persons with severe and persistent mental illness somewhat different from caring for persons who are physically ill or disabled.

Insights into the special issues of caring for patients with mental illness can be gained by reviewing the considerable body of research on the subject. Most of these issues, and therefore most of the research, are on the impact that caring has on the family. Much of the literature describes the experiences of caring, but in addition there are empirical studies on the relationship of family and patient to mental health professionals, the mental and physical effects of caring, and differences among caregivers based on their ethnicity. There are also a number of studies concerned with attempts to either reduce the burden of caring or to make caregivers more effective. This chapter reports on all of these issues and will make recommendations for the future. We have chosen to present separate sections on caring for young and middle-age adults—where caring usually relates to severe and persistent mental illnesses such as schizophrenia or bipolar affective illness (also called manic-depressive illness)—and on caring for older adults, where most of the caring focuses on dementia. (Caring for children with mental illness, while of critical importance, is beyond the scope of this chapter, although aspects of caring for children with mental retardation are discussed in chapter 2.)

We hope readers will reflect on what it is like to care for someone with severe mental illness, whose behavior and personality are distorted and with whom effective communication may be difficult and sometimes impossible. Interviews with parents of adult children with schizophrenia, conducted by Tuck et al. (1997), can give us a glimpse. One parent speaks of the pain, disappointment, and struggle. Another talks about the tentative nature of hope. What most have in common is summed up by one parent who said, "I guess you have to face the fact that parenting goes on forever" (120). If there is a simple, compelling phrase that captures the experience of those who care for loved ones with severe mental illness, it is the one used by Tuck and her colleagues: *endless caring.*

CARING FOR ADULTS WITH SEVERE AND PERSISTENT MENTAL ILLNESS

The Burden of "Endless Caring"

As we discuss caring, it is important to keep in mind who is doing it. A study by Hayden and Goldman (1996) on families of adults with mental retardation reiterates what many studies have shown: caring for mentally ill adults is typically provided by families. Although many family members might play a role, the majority of those who do are middle-aged women who generally have low levels of marital support and for whom caring is a lifelong role.

Objective and Subjective Burden. Researchers have paid much attention to the concept of burden in caring for the mentally ill (although, as we will note later, there is another side of the coin, because there are rewards as well). Caring produces both objective and subjective burdens—subjective referring to internal feelings related to being a caregiver; objective referring to observable consequences such as physical problems or limitations in social life. A study of seventy caregivers showed that the most frequent consequences of caring were emotional problems of the primary caregiver, disturbance of the caregiver's work, and disruption of the family household. The author concluded that more attention should be given to the needs of caregivers, both through educational sessions and direct attention to their physical and emotional health (Provencher, 1996). Another study, of partners of Vietnam veterans with post–traumatic stress disorder (PTSD), showed a reciprocal relationship between caregiver burden and the psychiatric pathology of the patient, with the worsening of one predicting a worsening of the other (Beckham, Lytle, and Feldman, 1996). Together, these two studies provide data enriching our understanding of Tuck's concept of endless caring and show that the effects of caring influence many aspects of daily life.

The interplay between patients and the people who care for them is highly variable. "Expressed emotion" (EE) is a concept that has been used to describe the quality of these interactions, and it usually means negative expressions by the caregiver, such as criticism of or hostility toward the patient. Caregiver EE is a negative factor in the course of schizophrenia (Brown, Birley, and Wing, 1972; Bebbington and Kuipers, 1994). It can make the endless caring inherent in the situation more difficult to bear.

A recent study (Bentsen et al., 1998) suggests that if factors predicting high EE could be identified, they might be modified, which in turn might stabilize a family's emotional status with resultant positive effects, including reduced rates of illness relapse by the patient. Noteworthy predictors of caregiver criticism in this study of relatives of recently hospitalized patients were the patient not having a paying job, more than three previous hospitalizations, and anxiety and depression. An unanticipated predictor of criticism was better cognitive functioning by the patient, suggesting that higher cognitive function may be misinterpreted as better ability to control symptoms. Predictors of caregiver hostility were lack of employment and more than three hospitalizations. It follows that detecting and treating depression and anxiety in patients with schizophrenia and keeping patients in paid employment whenever possible might reduce criticism and hostility, thus making endless caring a little easier.

Another helpful approach might be educational efforts to reduce relatives' unrealistic expectations, such as thinking that a patient's higher cognitive function would lessen the likelihood of relapse. Also, open discussion of relatives' inaccurate theories of the cause of mental illness, such as attributing psychiatric symptoms to moral weakness, might help lead to replacing these theories with an understanding of the genetic and biochemical bases of moods.

Relatives of recently hospitalized schizophrenia patients who had shown higher scores for burden of caring also perceived more deficits in patients' social functioning (Scazufca and Kuipers, 1996). The relatives' employment status was a predictor of EE status: working relatives had lower EE levels. Patients' psychopathology was not associated with EE levels or burden of care, however, suggesting that these elements are more dependent on relatives' perceptions rather than the patients' actual deficits. The clinical implications are that interventions directed at improving patients' social skills and at improving the ability of the family to deal constructively with the patient might favorably influence EE and patient outcomes.

Greenberg, Kim, and Greenley (1997) also found a subjective component to burden in their study of adult siblings. Although the well sibling's experience of burden of caring was consistently related to their ill sibling's actual symptomatology, the subjective component was clearly present; the study showed that those who viewed the troubling behavior as outside the patient's control experienced less burden. This strengthens the case that an educational approach directed at the subjective experiences of families might be beneficial. It also reminds us that the primary focus of treatment should be medication to control the patient's psychiatric symptoms, because that is likely to be the best course of action to help both patient and caregiver.

If professionals are to assist families in reducing the burden of caring for a mentally ill relative, families must be able to assess the degree of their burden accurately. But evidence suggests there are deficiencies in their ability to do so (Mueser et al., 1996). When degree of burden among relatives of patients with schizophrenia or bipolar illness was compared with how mental health professionals rated the amount of burden they believed relatives experienced, professionals underestimated the burden of delusions and lack of insight associated with mania. Since the professionals more accurately assessed the burden associated with these *symptoms* in schizophrenia, perhaps professionals need to assess burden associated with problem behaviors rather than burden associated with psychiatric diagnosis.

Health Consequences of Caring. Caring for individuals with mental illness can have unfavorable health consequences. McGilloway and Donnelly

(1997) reported that almost half of caregivers of long-stay psychiatric patients could be classified as "minor psychiatric cases" (according to the GHQ-12, a health questionnaire) and that they could possibly benefit from psychiatric treatment. An examination of the health and functioning of family members of patients with mental illness by Gallagher and Mechanic (1996) found that they had increased physician visits and hospital days, as well as activity limitations. Gender and kinship appear to be related to the health status of caregivers because living with either a mentally ill child or adult male relative increases health service utilization among non-mentally-ill household members. The trend toward deinstitutionalization of mental patients since the 1960s has increased the number of individuals faced with substantial caring responsibilities and has thereby created the "hidden costs" of caregiver health problems.

Another possible health consequence of caring is being a victim of abuse by a mentally ill relative. Vaddadi et al. (1997) reported that a majority of caregivers of hospitalized psychiatric patients experienced verbal abuse. Others (20%) suffered physical injury, with many of them reporting that they lived in fear of the patient. Physical abuse was more common when the diagnosis was schizophrenia or bipolar disorder than depression and, not surprisingly, was also related to the patients' current use of alcohol or cannabis. The array of health consequences associated with caring makes a strong argument for moving away from the traditional medical model to a broad approach that is directed toward both the patient and those who provide the caring.

Positive Aspects of Caring. With the negative consequences associated with caring for the mentally ill, it is heartening to learn that there are positive aspects as well. An example can be found among mothers of adult children with serious mental illness (Greenberg, 1995). A group of older mothers (over the age of fifty-five) indicated many areas in which mentally ill children provided them with assistance, such as doing chores, providing companionship, preparing meals, shopping, and providing care during times when the mother was ill. In many instances, mothers gained considerable emotional gratification from caring. In one instance, the mother said of her daughter, "She tells me all the time that I'm the best mother. It really feeds my ego, you know" (420).

Research has also shown that almost all caring relatives gain pleasure from, for example, seeing their ill relative happy (98%), seeing small improvements in the patient's condition (95%), seeing him or her well turned out (94%), receiving expressions of the relative's love (91%), and keeping the family member out of institutions (86%) (Grant et al., 1998). Again, vignettes provide a richness to the picture, such as a mother's comment about her adult daughter with multiple mental and physical disabilities: "She's got a great joy of life, and considering the amount of handicap she has, I mean, I've got nothing but admiration for her. I'm very proud of her" (264). It is not surprising that patient support of the caregiver is a predictor of family support, with the most prevalent form of patient support being symbolic, such as gift giving, expressing affection, and participating in family activities (Horwitz, Reinhard, and Howell-White, 1996).

Variations by Age, Race, and Ethnicity. So far we have spoken of those caring for mentally ill relatives in generalities, but common sense suggests that there are differences among them. This is indeed the case, with one important variable being age. Younger caregivers (those aged fifty-five or less) report significantly more unmet service needs that they regard as critical for those for whom they are caring (Hayden and Heller, 1997). Older caregivers (over fifty-five years of age) experience less personal burden and have lower expectations for services. Perhaps this difference is because younger caregivers have recently experienced a sharp drop off in school-based services available to mentally retarded individuals and have not yet had time to adjust to this.

Caring is also influenced by race and ethnicity. Black parents and siblings have at least as many caring responsibilities as white parents and siblings, yet they experience less caring burden (Horwitz and Reinhard, 1996). Stigma against mental illness was a strong predictor of burden, with black family members perceiving less of this than white families. Hispanic and African American caregivers tend to keep their ill relatives at home rather than looking to residential placement and see caring for someone with mental illness as a normative aspect of family life as opposed to a burden. Also, families in these two minority groups disagree with the assessments of mental health professionals more than do Euro-American families, being more likely to reject the medical model of mental illness and having higher expectations of their relative eventually being cured (Guarnaccia and Parra, 1995). Family caregivers in all three racial/ethnic groups experience substantially more burden when their relative is having prominent psychiatric symptoms (Stueve, Vine, and Struening, 1997). This provides additional support for the idea that prompt medication therapy is the most effective way to reduce burden in caregivers of acutely ill patients.

Benefits versus Burden? Analyzing the benefits versus burdens for families caring for a seriously ill relative is a complex and emotionally charged area. Family members have great difficulty characterizing their experiences as burdens or benefits. For example, a sister's personal experience with her brother's mental illness gave her a great passion for her career as a research psychiatrist, but she says she would hardly have chosen this life for him (Dixon, 1997). She wonders if professionals can appreciate the burdens of caring and encourages them to see family experiences as based on adaptation rather than pathology. She also observes that, while separating components of caring experiences such as burden and fear may be needed from a research perspective, in daily life they are experienced together. For example, her belief that her brother cannot control his symptoms may reduce her global burden, but her fears about what he may do in response to delusions that someone is trying to kill him increases her stress. She argues convincingly about the efficacy of psychoeducation for families and believes it has a proven place in managing many clinical situations.

Family Caregivers and Mental Health Professionals

Recent research and commentaries on caring for individuals with mental illness reflects an important shift in our thinking. We have moved away from seeing the family as the cause of mental illness to regarding family members as the patient's most valuable allies. To understand this more fully, we must examine the relationship between families and mental health professionals.

One of the recurring themes that Tuck et al. (1997) noted during lengthy interviews with a group of parents who were primary caregivers for adult children with schizophrenia was the mixed reactions of these parents to interactions with mental health professionals. On the one hand, the parents were desperate for information and grateful for a diagnosis that at least gave them something to hold on to. But they also felt frustration that diagnostic impressions could be subject to change and that confidentiality issues could make it difficult to get information they needed in order to help, such as whether their child was complying with medication. They greatly appreciated both information and support, as well as concern about how caring was affecting their lives.

Among the trends over the past few decades in the field of mental health (deinstitutionalization being the most notable one) has been family caregivers making their needs and expectations more clearly known to professionals. This has been highlighted by the growth of the National Alliance for the Mentally Ill (NAMI), an organization composed primarily of family members of individuals with severe and persistent mental illness. In 1993, NAMI conducted a survey of a little more than three thousand of its members to examine the services being used and how family members perceived them (Hatfield, Gearon, and Coursey, 1996); reflecting who does the caring for mentally ill adults, the respondents were mainly middle-aged women. Most of the patients (referred to by NAMI as consumers) had a diagnosis of schizophrenia or bipolar illness (57% and 21%, respectively). The three most frequently used services were medication (94%), individual therapy (69%), and hospitalization (61%). Medication (72%) and hospitalization (51%) received the highest ratings of being of considerable value, with residential care (50%) ranked third. Families placed greater value on office- and hospital-based services, while those considered to be essential to the community-based model, such as residential care and crisis care, were used less frequently.

A 1991 survey by a NAMI chapter showed that a significant minority of caregivers (34%) were dissatisfied with their contacts with mental health professionals (Biegel, Song, and Milligan, 1995). While this of course means that the majority (66%) were satisfied, there is room for improvement, and the results highlight the desire felt by many families to be included in the process of treatment. For example, only 28 percent were asked to help regulate or manage the patient's medication. Medication compliance is one of the major problems faced by family members who care for individuals with chronic mental illness, and this is an area where cooperation between family and professionals would be welcome and potentially helpful. Much remains to be done to strengthen relationships between family members and professionals.

Focus groups show that there is a desire for more information on the illness of the persons being cared for, such as the unexpected effects of new medications on the patient's behavior (Rose, 1998). Families want to express their opinions (such as hope for eventual improvement) without being judged and are particularly sensitive to criticism, such as admonishment for not recognizing the need for hospitalization sooner. Family members want easily available and prompt hospitalization during acute episodes, adequate community housing, and employment training for the patient. Perhaps the most important conclusion to be drawn from the literature on the relationship between caregivers and mental health professionals is that a dialogue is now underway, showing promise of an improved therapeutic partnership developing between these two groups.

Caring for the Caregiver

Caring for a relative of a patient with severe mental illness can be challenging. Relatives are often in conflict over whether to be more tolerant or more demanding. In the absence of professional guidance and support, they can easily undertake well-intentioned approaches that are ineffective or even counterproductive. For example, families of patients with obsessive-compulsive disorder who excessively accommodate to patients' rituals and behavior, modifying their own routines in dramatic ways (e.g., submitting to a patient's cleanliness rituals), may experience increased distress when such strategies do not reduce the level of behavior (Calvocoressi et al., 1995).

Psychoeducation and *family education* can assist families in coping with a mentally ill person (Solomon, 1996). Psychoeducation is a therapeutic approach developed originally for families of patients with schizophrenia as part of a comprehensive treatment package, including elements such as medication and outpatient clinical management, perhaps with social-skills training. Psychoeducation usually lasts several months and focuses on reducing negative expressed emotion (EE, discussed above), which can be related to psychotic relapse. Although psychoeducation appears to be cost-effective when compared with rehospitalization of the patient, and promotes strong relationships between families and professionals, the studies on it have limited generalizability because of stringent eligibility criteria on participating families. Some advocacy groups for the mentally ill are critical of psychoeducation because they find the association between EE and psychoeducation reminiscent of the outdated concept that mental illness is caused by the family. In contrast to psychoeducation, family education does not make the assumption that the family is being treated. As Solomon notes, family education is different from psychoeducation in that it focuses mainly on the needs of carers (i.e., families), not the needs of the ill relative, and emphasizes the strengths of the family, not its weaknesses. Family education is generally ten to twelve sessions long. Although there is evidence that families are more knowledgeable at the end of the program, and report less anxiety and distress, there is no evidence of an effect on rates of psychotic relapse. There is a need for both psychoeducation and family education, depending on the particular situation.

An even briefer counseling intervention of six one-hour counseling sessions has been reported for family members of schizophrenic patients (Bloch et al., 1995). A diverse array of themes emerged, covering issues such as grief and guilt, coping, dealing with dependency, and family issues such as attitudes toward mental illness. It seems clear that a broad array of interventions are needed.

Simple interventions can assist caring family members in getting into the medical care system. For example, to increase initial intake appointments at an inner-city mental health service for children, a thirty-minute telephone engagement was arranged with the child's caregiver, usually the mother or a foster parent (McKay, McCadam, and Gonzales, 1996). A significantly higher percentage of those involved in the extended telephone interaction kept their first appointments than did those receiving a more traditional, brief telephone interaction (73% vs. 45%). A good relationship between caregivers and professionals is beneficial, and particularly valuable if in place before crises occur.

An intriguing caring strategy was reported by Herman and Thompson (1995). Financially eligible families of developmentally disabled children in Michigan received a cash subsidy of $222 per month to purchase needed services. In addition, resources other than cash subsidy were used to provide babysitters (56% of families), respite care (40%), and adaptive equipment (42%). The cash subsidy was usually used for clothing (83%), general household expenses (61%), and educational aids and toys (63%). Although families regarded their basic needs as adequately met, they had few resources beyond those needed for basic survival. Cash subsidies have the value of being highly flexible, but they are not a replacement for formal professional services. There is an important role for both.

As interventions for caregivers continue to develop, we are likely to see specific interventions for specific diagnoses. For example, patients with borderline personality disorder—a diagnosis characterized by affect and impulse dyscontrol, dichotomous thinking (seeing others as either all good or all bad), and intolerance of aloneness—are regarded as demanding and difficult to treat, with frequent crises related to fears of abandonment. A psychoeducational group-treatment program has been developed, the intention being to enhance the ability of families to communicate with patients effectively and reduce their caring burden (Gunderson, Berkowitz, and Ruiz-Sancho, 1997). Guidelines are established—for example, to help maintain family routines and to avoid family members becoming defensive when criticized. The specificity of this approach may prove to be a useful model for other illnesses.

CARING FOR OLDER ADULTS WITH DEMENTIA

Dementia is not itself a disease but a group of symptoms that accompany certain diseases. It is the loss of intellectual abilities, thinking, remembering, and reasoning to such a severe degree that it interferes with a person's ability to function on a daily basis. Some of the well-known causes are Alzheimer disease, vascular dementia, Huntington's disease, Pick's disease, and Parkinson's disease. Dementia is included in this chapter because the greatest challenges in managing it are the behavioral problems associated with it.

The most common dementing illness is Alzheimer disease; according to the national Alzheimer's Association, it affects four million adults in the United States (Alzheimer's Association, 1998). It destroys memory, judgment, and the ability to communicate, often with profound changes in personality, mood, and behavior. This progressive, degenerative disease can span twenty years or more, with individuals eventually being unable to care for themselves. Mace and Rabins titled their family guide for caring for people with Alzheimer disease and related disorders *The 36-Hour Day*—an apt way to describe the reality of caring for older adults with dementia.

Besides the four million people afflicted with Alzheimer disease, 19 million caregivers are affected. By the year 2050, it is estimated, there will be 14 million people in the United States with dementia (Alzheimer's Association, 1998). At the same time, however, the pool of potential caregivers will decrease. According to the Institute for Health and Aging at the University of California, San Francisco, in 1990 the ratio of people aged from fifty to sixty-four to people aged more than eighty-five was eleven to one: by 2050, this ratio will be four to one (Institute for Health and Aging, 1996).

The Impact of Caring

A considerable amount of research on dementia focuses on the impact of caring—primarily on the negative impacts on the family caregiver. Rapp and Reynolds (1999) have summarized this research, reporting that studies show both cross-sectional and prospective associations between caring workload demands and increased psychological distress for the caregiver, particularly depression and anxiety. They report that the challenges associated with caring for someone with dementing illnesses—such as dealing with incontinence, severe functional impairment, hallucinations, delusions, agitation, wandering, aggressiveness, and the need for constant supervision—are associated with high levels of caregiver strain. And, as the demands increase or become more intrusive, caregivers may experience restrictions on their social and leisure activities; a loss of privacy; conflicts with other role demands at work and home; increased conflict with family members; financial strain; feelings of guilt, anger, frustration, helplessness, and grief; and physical exhaustion. Rapp and Reynolds also note that the negative psychiatric effects of caring for a demented family member can become chronic. Psychiatric morbidity in caregivers is most consistently linked to problem behaviors of the patient, low income, poor self-rated health, increased perceived stress, and decreased life satisfaction.

The extensive pressure on caregivers of persons with Alzheimer disease (spouses, children, siblings, extended family, and friends) often appear as distress and depression (Teri, 1997), which are highly correlated with behavioral dysfunction of Alzheimer patients and their depression-related behaviors. Agitation, particularly physical aggression, may affect a caregiver even more than a patient's depression or memory loss (Victoroff, Mack, and Nielson, 1998). Some question whether caregivers are depressed or experiencing grief, suggesting that the depression so frequently described may not be as severe or clinically significant as previously thought (Walker and Pomeroy, 1996). It may be anticipatory grief engendered by the losses they are experiencing and further losses they expect to experience.

Caring for someone with dementia would logically also seem to place the caregiver at risk for physical health problems, but the evidence on this is less clear than for severe and persistent mental illness. In a comprehensive review of physical health outcomes in dementia caregivers—including determinations of medication use, chronic physical illnesses, acute illnesses, health care utilization, and immune and cardiovascular functioning—few variables emerged as consistent predictors of the burden of caring for demented persons. Financial strain, high psychological distress, low social support, and high levels of cognitive impairment in patients, however, did seem to be associated with poorer health status in caregivers (Schulz et al., 1995). In addition to these four variables, patient behavior problems (e.g., inappropriate aggressiveness, and incontinence) are also associated with physical health problems, according to research reported by Rapp and Reynolds (1999).

The impacts on caregivers from caring for demented patients appear to be influenced by race, ethnicity, and culture. In a detailed review and analysis of empirical research that has examined the impact of race, culture, and ethnicity on the dementia caregiving experience, ten of the twelve studies reviewed compared black and white caregivers, one looked at the differences between black and Hispanic caregivers, and one focused on white and Hispanic caregivers (Connell and Gibson, 1997). The non-white caregivers reported lower levels of stress, burden, and depression; they also endorsed more strongly held beliefs about filial support; and they were more likely to use prayer, faith, or religion as coping mechanisms. Compared with white caregivers, nonwhite (black and Hispanic) caregivers of demented family members are less likely to be a spouse and more likely to be an adult child, friend, or other family member. If a caregiver is of advanced old age, this can be a factor in the caring relationship. The prevalence of dementia among persons aged sixty-five and older is between 5 percent and 10 percent; among those aged eighty-five and older, it is in the range of 25 percent to 48 percent. Because the prevalence among very old persons is so high, married couples who are of advanced old age are at risk for both members experiencing cognitive problems. Unfortunately, demented patients with cognitively impaired spouses utilize fewer community resources and experience difficulty with medication compliance more often than those with cognitively normal spousal caregivers (Boucherl, Renvall, and Jackson, 1996). Cognitive disability in both members of an elderly couple represents a particularly difficult challenge in caring.

Caring as a Positive Experience

Very little has been written acknowledging the positive aspects and outcomes of caring for demented persons (although as noted in chapter 10, no completely satisfactory ways to measure the outcomes of caring have yet been developed). What are the positive aspects of caring for a demented loved one? In *Helping Yourself Help Others: A Book for Caregivers,* Carter and Golant (1994) devoted a chapter to "finding fulfillment," not wanting to leave the impression that caregiving is an onerous task with few rewards. Participants in their CARE-NET study said that, despite its difficulty, caring for a cognitively impaired elderly relative fostered pleasure, love, personal growth, family closeness, and fulfillment. Through personal stories, caregivers related how the experience changed their lives for the good: becoming more sensitive, compassionate, and patient; learning to listen more; developing a sense of humor; improving attitudes, values, and relationships; having a better understanding of themselves; and gaining a new respect for life.

Appreciating and finding pleasure in caring seems to be more likely among caregivers who are in good health (Gold et al., 1995). The availability of greater numbers of family members and friends who provide social and emotional support also increases the positive outcomes of caregiving. Gender also plays a role: although in this study women experienced higher levels of burden than men, they were able to find more aspects of caregiving enjoyable.

Because dementia caregiving usually involves family, it is noteworthy that the literature addresses the positive impact on adolescent relationships. A study by Beach (1997) focused on adolescents who were either a child, a grandchild, or a niece or nephew of a person with Alzheimer disease or related disorder who was being cared for by the adolescent's immediate family. The results showed increased sibling sharing, greater empathy for older adults, and significant mother-adolescent bonding.

Caring for the Caregivers

For several decades, efforts have been made to assess the nature and extent of distress caregivers endure in caring for the seriously mentally ill. More recently, researchers have turned their attention to the identification and effects of coping techniques used by family caregivers and to the impact of supportive services.

Caregivers use different strategies to help their situations, and sometimes they have more than one way to deal with the burden of caring for demented family members. For many, accepting their situation, seeking information, and seeking social supports seem to be effective coping strategies (Almberg, Grafström, and Winblad, 1997) that buffer the adverse impact of caregiving (Rapp and Reynolds, 1999). Caregivers who engage in active support-seeking behaviors, such as requesting help and guiding their helpers, report being healthier, happier with their lives, and less depressed; they receive more benefits from caring than less socially assertive caregivers (Rapp et al., 1998).

There are a variety of services that can have a positive impact on the person afflicted with dementia. One example is participation in support groups such as those sponsored by local chapters of the Alzheimer's Association. Another example is the training of caregivers so that they cope more effectively—a service that can delay institutionalization of persons with dementia. An eight-year survival analysis (Brodaty, Gresham, and Luscombe, 1997) indicated that patients with mild to moderate dementia stayed at home significantly longer and tended to live longer if their caregivers received a structured, residential, intensive ten-day training program, coupled with follow-ups and telephone conferences over a period of twelve months. In a randomized, controlled intervention study involving more than two hundred spouse caregivers of persons with Alzheimer disease, the caregivers were provided with six sessions of individual and family counseling and were required to join support groups (Mittelman et al., 1996). This program of counseling and support substantially increased the time spouses were able to care at home for their loved one with dementia, particularly during the early to middle stages of the disease, when nursing home placement is generally least appropriate. In a longitudinal treatment/control study (Mittelman et al., 1995) that examined the effects of a comprehensive support program on depression, caregivers of patients with Alzheimer disease received a psychosocial intervention program consisting of individual and family counseling, continuous availability of ad hoc counseling, and support-group participation. In the first year after intake, the control group became increasingly more depressed, whereas the treatment group remained stable, suggesting that long-term social support can have a significant impact on depression in caregivers.

Adult day centers are a growing national resource that can serve elderly individuals who live at home, providing therapeutic benefit to both patients and those who care for them (Reifler et al., 1997; 1999). The use of these centers by caregivers of dementia patients results in lower levels of caregiving-related stress and better psychological well-being for caregivers when compared with controls. In a study comparing users to nonusers, findings for one year showed that the caregiver group that used adult day services had significantly lower scores on overload and depression than the control group (Zarit et al., 1998).

SUMMARY AND RECOMMENDATIONS

In this chapter, we have considered the burdens and rewards that families experience in caring for patients who have severe and persistent mental illness. We have also looked at the challenges that mental health professionals face in caring for family caregivers. The key findings from research on these issues are summarized below, accompanied by recommendations for improving the quality of caring.

Caring for adults with severe and persistent mental illness is provided primarily by middle-aged women who face caring as a lifelong task, often with little help from other family members. They are very diverse in terms of the attitudes, needs, and details of their caring experience. Thus, a variety of approaches will be necessary to meet their needs, including better communication with professionals, psychoeducational and family educational opportunities, and perhaps even cash subsidies. Cultural and diagnosis-specific approaches need further development.

The concept that the family is the cause of mental illness is outdated and counterproductive; it also perpetuates widely held misconceptions about mental illness. One way to counteract this misconception is through legislation mandating coverage of mental illness by insurers at a level equivalent to coverage for physical illness—often referred to as parity. Currently, most insurance plans have limitations on annual outpatient and inpatient treatment that do not apply to physical illness. These limitations have no medical justification.

Assisting those who are caring for the mentally ill requires moving beyond the concept of burden and recognizing that the caregiver and patient form a dyad. No one can doubt the notion of "endless caring," but there are opportunities for the caring person and patient to define how they will deal with the situation in which they find themselves. Professionals must provide the services that they alone can do, such as medical management, but they must also respect and understand the knowledge and needs of the patient and caregiver as well.

Better understanding is needed of how individuals adapt coping behaviors to a changing situation; for example, caring for someone with a progressive disease, such as Alzheimer's, that is incurable. This understanding will have to differentiate between men and women caregivers; the sexes may differ in their approaches to caring.

Older adults with dementia should remain in familiar surroundings in their own community. Attention must be given to the emotional, intellectual, and physical needs of both patients and caregivers. Adult day services and home health care are examples of programs that help to achieve this. A systematic collaborative approach of government, community, family, and health care is necessary.

ACKNOWLEDGMENTS

The authors of this chapter wish to thank Diane Joyner and Marsha Honeycutt for their assistance.

REFERENCES

Almberg, B., Grafström, M., and Winblad, B. (1997). Major strain and coping strategies as reported by family members who care for aged demented relatives. *Journal of Advanced Nursing* 26: 683–91.

Alzheimer's Association (1998). <http: //www.alz.org/facts/index.html>, September 28.

Beach, D. L. (1997). Family caregiving: The positive impact on adolescent relationships. *Gerontologist* 37(2): 233–38.

Bebbington, P., and Kuipers, L. (1994). The predictive utility of expressed emotion in schizophrenia: An aggregate analysis. *Psychological Medicine* 24: 707–18.

Beckham, J. C., Lytle, B. L., and Feldman, M. E. (1996). Caregiver burden in partners of Vietnam war veterans with posttraumatic stress disorder. *Journal of Consulting and Clinical Psychology* 64(5): 1068–72.

Bentsen, H., Notland, T. H., Boye, B., Munkvold, O.-G., Bjørge, Lersbryggen, A. B., Uren, G., Oskarsson, K. H., Berg-Larsen, R., Lingjærde, O., and Malt, U. F. (1998). Criticism and hostility in relatives of patients with schizophrenia or related psychoses: Demographic and clinical predictors. *Acta Psychiatrica Scandinavica* 97: 76–85.

Biegel, D. E., Song, L., and Milligan, S. E. (1995). A comparative analysis of family caregivers' perceived relationships with mental health professionals. *Psychiatric Services* 46(5): 477–82.

Bloch, S., Szmukler, G. I., Herrman, H., Benson, A., and Colussa, S. (1995). Counseling caregivers of relatives with schizophrenia: Themes, interventions, and caveats. *Family Process* 34: 413–25.

Boucher, L., Renvall, M. J., and Jackson, J. E. (1996). Cognitively impaired spouses as primary caregivers for demented elderly people. *Journal of the American Geriatric Society* 44: 828–31.

Brodaty, H., Gresham, M., and Luscombe, G. (1997). The Prince Henry Hospital dementia caregivers training programme. *International Journal of Geriatric Psychiatry* 12: 183–92.

Brown, G. W., Birley, J. L. T., and Wing, J. K. (1972). Influence of family life on the course of schizophrenic disorders: A replication. *British Journal of Psychiatry* 121: 241–58.

Calvocoressi, L., Lewis, B., Harris, M., Trufan, S. J., Goodman, W. K., McDougle, C. J., Price, L. H. (1995). Family accommodation in obsessive-compulsive disorder. *American Journal of Psychiatry* 152(3): 441–43.

Carter, R., and Golant, S. K. (1994). *Helping Yourself Help Others: A Book for Caregivers.* New York: Times Books.

Connell, C. M., and Gibson, G. D. (1997). Racial, ethnic, and cultural differences in dementia caregiving: Review and analysis. *Gerontologist* 37(3): 355–64.

Dixon, L. (1997). The next generation of research: Views of a sibling-psychiatrist-researcher. *American Journal of Orthopsychiatry* 67(2): 242–48.

Gallagher, S. K., and Mechanic, D. (1996). Living with the mentally ill: Effects on the health and functioning of other household members. *Social Science Medicine* 42(12): 1691–701.

Gold, D. P., Cohen, C., Shulman, K., Zucchero, C., Andres, D., and Etezadi, J. (1995). Caregiving and dementia: Predicting negative and positive outcomes for caregivers. *International Journal of Aging and Human Development* 41(3): 183–201.

Grant, G., Ramcharan, P., McGrath, M., Nolan, M., and Keady, J. (1998). Rewards and gratifications among family caregivers: Towards a refined model of caring and coping. *Journal of Intellectual Disability Research* 42(1): 58–71.

Greenberg, J. S. (1995). The other side of caring: Adult children with mental illness as supports to their mothers in later life. *Social Work* 40(3): 414–23.

Greenberg, J. S., Kim, H. W., and Greenley, J. R. (1997). Factors associated with subjective burden in siblings of adults with severe mental illness. *American Journal of Orthopsychiatry* 67(2): 231–41.

Guarnaccia, P. J., and Parra, P. (1996). Ethnicity, social status, and families' experiences of caring for a mentally ill family member. *Community Mental Health Journal* 32(3): 243–60.

Gunderson, J. G., Berkowitz, C., and Ruiz-Sancho, A. (1997). Families of borderline patients: A psychoeducational approach. *Bulletin of the Menninger Clinic* 61(4): 446–57.

Hatfield, A. B., Gearon, J. S., and Coursey, R. D. (1996). Family members ratings of the use and value of mental health services: Results of a national NAMI survey. *Psychiatric Services* 47(8): 825–31.

Hayden, M. F., and Goldman, J. (1996). Families of adults with mental retardation: Stress levels and need for services. *Social Work* 41(6): 657–67.

Hayden, M. F., and Heller, T. (1997). Support, problem-solving/coping ability, and personal burden of younger and older caregivers of adults with mental retardation. *Mental Retardation* 35(5): 364–72.

Herman, S. E., and Thompson, L. (1995). Families' perceptions of their resources for caring for children with developmental disabilities. *Mental Retardation* 33(2): 73–83.

Horwitz, A. V., and Reinhard, S. C. (1995). Ethnic differences in caregiving duties and burdens among parents and siblings of persons with severe mental illnesses. *Journal of Health and Social Behavior* 36: 138–50.

Horwitz, A. V., Reinhard, S. C., and Howell-White, S. (1996). Caregiving as reciprocal exchange in families with seriously mentally ill members. *Journal of Health and Social Behavior* 37: 149–62.

Institute for Health and Aging, University of California, San Francisco (1996).

Chronic Care in America: A 21st Century Challenge. Princeton, NJ: Robert Wood Johnson Foundation.

Mace, N. L., and Rabins, P. V. (1999). *The 36-Hour Day: A Family Guide to Caring for Persons with Alzheimer Disease, Related Dementing Illnesses, and Memory Loss in Later Life.* 3rd ed. Baltimore, MD: Johns Hopkins University Press.

McGilloway, S., and Donnelly, M. (1997). The experience of caring for former long-stay psychiatric patients. *British Journal of Clinical Psychology* 36: 149–51.

McKay, M. M., McCadam, K., and Gonzales, J. J. (1996). Addressing the barriers to mental health services for inner city children and their caretakers. *Community Mental Health Journal* 32(4): 353–61.

Mittelman, M. S., Ferris, S. H., Shulman, E., Steinberg, G., Ambinder, A., Mackell, J. A., and Cohen, J. (1995). A comprehensive support program: Effect on depression in spouse-caregivers of AD patients. *Gerontologist* 35(6): 792–802.

Mittelman, M. S., Ferris, S. H., Shulman, E., Steinberg, G., and Levin, B. (1996). A family intervention to delay nursing home placement of patients with Alzheimer disease: A randomized controlled trial. *Journal of the American Medical Association* 276(21): 1725–31.

Mueser, K. T., Webb, C., Pfeiffer, M., Gladis, M., and Levinson, D. F. (1996). Family burden of schizophrenia and bipolar disorder: Perceptions of relatives and professionals. *Psychiatric Services* 47(5): 507–11.

Peabody, F. W. (1927). The care of the patient. *Journal of the American Medical Association* 88: 877–82.

Provencher, H. L. (1996). Objective burden among primary caregivers of persons with chronic schizophrenia. *Journal of Psychiatric and Mental Health Nursing* 3: 181–87.

Rapp, S. R., and Reynolds, D. L. (1999). Families, social support, and caregiving. In W. R. Hazzard, J. P. Blass, W. H. Ettinger, J. B. Walter, and J. G. Ouslander, eds., *Principles of Geriatric Medicine and Gerontology*, pp. 333–43. New York: McGraw-Hill.

Rapp, S. R., Shumaker, S., Schmidt, S., Naughton, M., and Anderson, R. (1998). Social resourcefulness: Its relationship to social support and wellbeing among caregivers of dementia victims. *Aging Mental Health* 2(1): 40–48.

Reifler, B. V., Cox, N. J., Jones, B. N., Rushing, J., and Yates, K. (1999). Service use and financial performance in a replication program on adult day centers. *American Journal of Geriatric Psychiatry* 7(2): 98–107.

Reifler, B. V., Henry, R. S., Rushing, J., Yates, K., Cox, N. J., Bradham, D. D., and McFarlane, M. (1997). Financial performance among adult day centers: Results of a national demonstration program. *Journal of the American Geriatric Society* 45: 146–53.

Rose, L. (1998). Benefits and limitations of professional-family interactions: The family perspective. *Archives of Psychiatric Nursing* 12(3): 140–47.

Scazufca, M., and Kuipers, E. (1996). Links between expressed emotion and burden of care in relatives of patients with schizophrenia. *British Journal of Psychiatry* 168: 580–87.

Schulz, R., O'Brien, A. T., Bookwala, J., and Fleissner, K. (1995). Psychiatric and physical morbidity effects of dementia caregiving: Prevalence, correlates, and causes. *Gerontologist* 35(6): 771–91.

Solomon, P. (1996). Moving from psychoeducation to family education for families of adults with serious mental illness. *Psychiatric Services* 47(12): 1364–70.

Stueve, A., Vine, P., and Struening, E. L. (1997). Perceived burden among caregivers of adults with serious mental illness: Comparison of black, Hispanic, and white families. *American Journal of Orthopsychiatry* 67(2): 199–209.

Teri, L. (1997). Behavior and caregiver burden: Behavioral problems in patients with Alzheimer's disease and its association with caregiver distress. *Alzheimer Disease and Associated Disorders* 11 supplement 4: S35–S38.

Tuck, I., du Mont, P., Evans, G., and Shupe, J. (1997). The experience of caring for an adult child with schizophrenia. *Archives of Psychiatric Nursing* 11(3): 118–25.

Vaddadi, K. S., Soosai, E., Gilleard, C. J., and Adlard, S. (1997). Mental illness, physical abuse, and burden of care on relatives: A study of acute psychiatric admission patients. *Acta Psychiatrica Scandinavica* 95: 313–17.

Victoroff, J., Mack, W. J., and Nielson, K. A. (1998). Psychiatric complications of dementia: Impact on caregivers. *Dementia and Geriatric Cognitive Disorders* 9: 50–55.

Walker, R. J., and Pomeroy, E. (1996). Depression or grief? The experience of caregivers of people with dementia. *Health and Social Work* 21(4): 247–54.

Zarit, S. H., Stephens, M. A. P., Townsend, A., and Greene, R. (1998). Stress reduction for family caregivers: Effects of adult day care use. *Journal of Gerontology* 53B(5): S267–S277.

II

THE PROVISION OF CARING

4

A History of Caring in Medicine

JOEL D. HOWELL, M.D., PH.D.

For as long as we can go back in time, people have cared for one another. People have cared for their children and their parents, for their loved ones, for their friends, for others whom they knew not. People have cared for human beings found alone and in pain; they have cared for people at home and within institutions. Care, in all of these settings, involves *caring*—listening, understanding, empathy, compassion, counseling, and providing emotional support. Caring is an element of basic human decency, and most people would agree that it is part of being a good person.

At times, society has held some people responsible for care. Sometimes the responsibility for it has been assigned to one person, at other times to larger groups. Sometimes the differentiation has been made on the basis of sex, sometimes on the basis of specific training. Health care providers have always had a special relationship with those people whom they serve.

What it means to provide health care has certainly changed over the years, both in context and in content. To speak about *caring* and *curing* as though they were two distinct concepts would have made little sense to an early-nineteenth-century American. Each would have been one side of the same coin, impossible to separate without doing away with both. Today, the fact that we can make the separation at all says much about the ways in which our conceptualization of the role of the healer has changed.

Nominally, health care providers have always been charged with caring for those to whom they minister. For such providers, caring has at times been part of a larger set of professional responsibilities. Yet the titles and functions attached to those health care providers have changed over the years. So, too, caring has meant very different things over the years. Those meanings have always been embedded in a social and cultural context that defined what was good and what was possible. In this chapter, we explore the various meanings of caring over time, focusing our attention on the United States of America.

CARING IN EARLY AMERICA

Family and Community Responsibilities

First in the colonies and later in the early years of the United States, most settlers lived their lives in a world of small communities, connected only by tenuous linkages. Crude trails and modest dirt roads connecting villages were often impassable for months at a time due to rain, mud, or snow. If a town was on the ocean or a navigable river, waterborne transportation was often more reliable than going by road, at least when the water was free of ice. Mail service was erratic at best. Groups of people thus tended to be geographically isolated from each other, and the essential basis of social organization lay within each community.

Within a village, the key organizational component was the family, which constituted the primary unit for almost every interaction among community members, whether social, religious, or a matter of business. Among the duties of families was care for people in need of assistance due to illness and suffering. The family's responsibilities did not include only blood relatives: the head of the household was also responsible for the care of the family servants, should they become ill (Demos, 1970). Families also held the duty of caring for their parents and grandparents as they aged and became infirm or frail. However, even in the small communities of the early United States, this duty seems not to have been universally accepted. Some colonial husbands felt the need to write wills specifically designed to ensure that their widows would receive proper care by making bequests available to children only on the condition that they fulfill the appropriate filial duties of caring for their aging parent or parents (Demos, 1970).

While being a member of a family was important, to be sure, a person's responsibilities to her or his community were taken with the same measure of seriousness as were responsibilities to the family. Caring was not only a family responsibility but a communal obligation. The community at large took on the task of providing for the care of those who could not care for themselves. Sometimes the town would send people who needed medical care to live in households as "patients" to be cared for by members of the community who were known to be skilled in the practice of medicine, whether or not those people had any formal training as physicians. To eliminate some of the cost for households that agreed to take in a sick person, the community might agree to bear the financial responsibility for the care that was provided (Demos, 1970).

Perhaps the most famous example of communal responsibility for care occurred in the early days of the Republic, in 1822, on the isolated island of Mackinac, northern Michigan. There, on a bright June day, a shotgun was accidentally discharged into the side of a French fur trapper, Alexis St. Martin. Although St. Martin survived the initial episode, the wound into his stomach did not heal. When St. Martin could no longer take care of himself or provide for his family, he was cared for in the home of an early American physician, William Beaumont, at community expense, in the small village on the desolate island. Over the next few years, Beaumont moved from caring for St. Martin to studying him, putting various types of food directly into St. Martin's stomach and observing the actions of the digestive juices. Beaumont thus may have been the first person in the United States to undertake physiological research.

Although the combination of caring with scientific study was remarkable, such instances of the community caring for an individual were not unusual. Hospitals, which existed in only a few cities, were places that would never be entered by a respectable member of society—places where only the poor and destitute would ever go to receive care. In any event, for almost all Americans, hospitals were not readily available. Consequently, people who could not care for themselves and did not have a family capable of providing for their care would either be cared for in households within the community or not at all. Because the responsibility for care was held to belong to the entire community, the resources that could (not to mention *should*) be brought to bear for care of the ill and destitute were far more available than they were in later periods in U.S. history.

The general sense of community obligation came partly from ideas about what commitments people were thought to owe to their fellow human beings. Communities judged people by their fulfillment of duty. Characteristics such as "individuality" or "self-reliance" were not desirable attributes for a person in early American society. Ideal citizens would carry out their social obligations above all else—obligations that were important for men as well as women. Both sexes shared in the communal responsibility for care. They could do so in part because definitions of success allowed it to be so. A man's identity was a function not of his individual accomplishments but of what he owed to the community (Rotundo, 1993). His social standing was largely determined by the circumstances of his birth, not by what he accomplished. Men were not driven to work hard outside of the household in order to become a success. But this was soon to change, and change in a way that made a clear differentiation between the sexes with respect to who was responsible for care.

Women, Men, and Caring Responsibilities

Looking back over the twentieth century, one can see a movement toward increasing gender equality—a movement that in large part developed in response to an earlier, general, widespread belief that, while men should go out into the workplace, a woman's place was in the home—that women had some sort of poorly defined, ineffable affinity with the domestic scene. One might be tempted to see these as natural beliefs that had always existed. Such was not the case. These ideas came into existence during a definable historical period.

During the early nineteenth century, what the social historian E. Anthony Rotundo (1993) has called the "communal" form of manhood, in which men lived in a world defined by their birth and their community, was eclipsed by "self-made manhood," in which men came to be defined by their achievements in the workplace. This new definition of manhood detracted from the traditional communal value given to caring provided by men. Men were now driven by aggression, rivalry, and ambition. The task of work increasingly took them out of the home and the household, out of the community, into factories or cities, and thus made them unavailable for tasks around the house.

As a consequence, the need to care for members of the community or the family became a task increasingly left to women. As men gave in to "selfish passions" outside the home, women came to be seen as those most responsible for the common good—for caring. Women were held to be innately different from men; they were the spiritual and moral center of not only the family but of society at large. Thus was created the doctrine of separate spheres—the idea that men were destined for the workplace, the "world," while women were best suited to carry out the duties of the home. This sex-based differentiation had and continues to have profound consequences for our ideas about who ought to be the primary caregivers for those in need.

If women's place was in the home, it followed that home care for the ill (and that was where most ill people were cared for) was a "natural" female function. From this arose the idea, so dramatically expressed by the nursing pioneer Florence Nightingale, that "Every woman is a nurse"; she went on to explain that every woman must "at some time or other of her life . . . have charge of somebody's health" (Nightingale, 1860 [1969]: 4). Indeed, as the historian Emily Abel (1991, 2000) has well explained, the experience of nursing, of caring for the ill, came to be a dominant influence on most women's lives. Women cared not only for frail and ill older persons—people at the end of a long life—but also for those who fell ill as infants and children (and often died). Women cared for others in settings that were both dangerous and unpleasant. Women cared not only for members of their immediate families but also for extended-family members, sometimes, if necessary, in distant cities. A woman was always at risk to be called upon to care for someone, no matter what the current status of her life. An 1837 book of advice for young ladies warned them: "You may be called upon at any moment to attend upon your parents, your brothers, your sisters, or your companions" (Farrar, 1837: 57). No duty was held to be more important. While caring for the sick, a woman was expected to give herself over completely and unquestioningly to the task. Women were thought to be particularly appropriate and naturally attuned to care for children, their abilities flowing naturally from the experience of maternity (Murphy, 1991).

Women also took the lead in working to improve conditions for care of people outside the home, especially women and children, and some wanted to expand the concept of motherhood to include all of society, based on the idea that the innate, feminine attributes of women would benefit almost every sphere of the social world, particularly by contributing to organizations devoted to improving the plight of the poor, dependent, and sick members of society (Baker, 1984). Women were thought to have an elevated moral status, one that enabled them to uphold key values in caring not only for the ill but also for the well, not only for their family but also for society at large.

CARING AND THE NINETEENTH-CENTURY PHYSICIAN

Although today we think of physicians as central to health care, we do not usually see the physician as devoting as much energy to caring as to, say, the careful evaluation of evidence from medical technologies and laboratories. Where did physicians fit into the nineteenth-century world when medical technologies and laboratories were absent or very limited?

Although it was often difficult for patient and physician to meet (a situation discussed below), when physicians did make it to the bedside in the nineteenth-century United States, they were more likely to play a role in caring for their patients than were those of the next century.

The Social Status of Physicians

Compassion, listening, counseling, support, and giving of time and oneself are the hallmarks of caring. It is not surprising that these elements of caring are most easily to be found in members of the person's immediate family, religious group, or community. In the nineteenth century and until more recent times, physicians also undertook such caring. Perhaps the most important reason was that being a physician was not a particularly high-status occupation throughout most of the nineteenth century and well into the twentieth. (The truly elite professions, places where the best and the brightest might wish to go, tended to be the law and the clergy.)

Life as a physician was difficult, insecure, and not very financially rewarding. Incomes were unlikely to be significantly higher than those of the surrounding townspeople. Physicians often held down two jobs; in addition to working as a physician, the doctor might also work a farm or run a pharmacy. Such jobs led physicians to interact on a regular basis with many members of the community, often in settings where the physician was likely to be seen in the same position on the social scale as the people he or she served; they lived, worked, prayed, and played together. Even as the revolution in medical education started to change these relationships, physicians were still given careful advice on how important it was to fit into the community: how to behave, how to dress, with whom to associate (Howell, 1997). The young physician seeking a place to start a practice was advised:

> By all means seek to locate in a community to which you are suited; that will be congenial as a place to live in, and in which you are likely to get business and be useful to your fellow-beings, and also to earn a living for your self. Remember that unpopular opinions in politics or religion injure, and that, all else equal, you will be more likely to succeed in a section where your views, habits, and tastes are naturally in harmony with the bulk of the people, morally, socially, and politically. (Cathell, 1890: 3)

With fewer boundaries between the ordinary citizenry and the professions—not only physicians but most other professions, too—physicians may have been more inclined than those in some other callings to regard caring as part of their mission. In order to be close, physicians and patients needed to speak the same language, both literally and metaphorically, and most tended to do so.

The Theory and Practice of Medicine

Moreover, nineteenth-century medical theories tended to promote this sort of caring. In contrast to the understanding at the end of the twentieth century, sickness was not ascribed to a specific cause such as an identifiable microorganism or a deranged bodily part. Rather, sickness was a condition affecting the entire human organism. Although there was a good deal of "scientific" knowledge to be learned in order to be an excellent physician, the epistemological basis of that knowledge held that the key role of the physician was to select from the entire range of possibilities the proper drug in the proper dose to treat a specific individual; universal knowledge of the available drugs could serve as a guide, but the therapy for each person needed to be individualized. There was, for example, no specific microorganism to be treated. Each person was unique, each person's temperament would play a key role not only in making a diagnosis but also in guiding the hand of the physician in recommending appropriate therapy.

Thus, getting to know the patient was an essential part of medical practice. What was the family history? Was this person easily angered? Or somewhat slow and quiet? If one did not know the patient well, one could not make efficient use of the available therapeutic armamentarium. As the medical historian Charles E. Rosenberg has noted, "A physician who knew a family's constitutional idiosyncrasies was necessarily a better practitioner for a family than one who enjoyed no such insight—or even one who hailed from a different climate, for it was assumed that both the action of drugs and reaction of patients varied with season and geography" (Rosenberg, 1979: 11). Moreover, physicians treated patients in the home and thus were familiar with that patient's family and specific living conditions. This familiarity emphasized the importance of individual and family characteristics, beliefs, culture, financial circumstances, and other dimensions particular to the patient and enhanced the physician's capacity to be an effective caregiver. Perhaps compassion was easier to come by when patients were seen in context and when the context was similar for patient and physician (and, in relevant situations, the family caregiver). Because a local physician knew well the patient and his or her family and environs, a physician from afar, no matter how well trained, was by definition less competent. (This epistemology was another reason hospitals were seen as irrelevant to much of medical care, for if disease were seen as part of its local context in a hospital, it could not be the same as a disease in the community.) Seeing the patient in her or his home served to emphasize the importance of a local and specific understanding of disease to the patient and physician and family, and may have promoted an element of caring and compassion.

As we begin the twenty-first century, we may be tempted to see nineteenth-century therapies and therapeutic epistemologies as far-fetched at best and somewhat silly at worst. But we should try to avoid this perspective for at least two important reasons. First, such thinking does us little good if we wish to use history to inform present-day policymaking. History may be most useful to us insofar as it provides a model for understanding change. Obviously, we cannot use facts and ideas unavailable to people in the nineteenth century as a means of explaining why they behaved as they did. If we wish to understand change, we can do so only by understanding the facts as they existed at the time of the events we wish to explain, not later. A second reason can quite simply be suggested by contemplating how ridiculous many present-day therapies are likely to appear a century from today.

No matter what physicians' ideas were in the nineteenth century and the early part of the twentieth century, the fact is that physicians, because of practical difficulties, were often not available when a person fell ill. The country was overwhelmingly rural, well-trained physicians were few, and transportation was difficult. Absent the telephone, one could not call the doctor's office to see if the physician was available to see a patient. Communication was usually done directly by a person traveling on horseback or on foot. Thus, if the sick person was on a farm, a not uncommon occurrence, contacting the physician in a village required that a healthy person be away from work on the farm for some time. It could easily take an entire day for the messenger to go into town, find a note at the doctor's home indicating where he or she had gone, go out to that new location, and accompany the doctor back to the farm. The costs in terms of lost work were high and would be incurred only if it was judged that the value of the patient being seen by a trained physician equaled those costs, which was often not the case.

Even if a physician was readily available, medical ideas were often portrayed as having little to add to what was necessary to care for an ill person. Far less status was given to the scientific basis of the field than today.

As Gunn's *Domestic Medicine*, a popular guide to health care, put it, "For the common and useful purposes of mankind, the refined fripperies and hair-drawn theories of mere science, are of no use whatever; indeed they have never had much other effect, than to excite a stupid admiration of men who pretended to know more than the mass of mankind" (Gunn, 1830 [1986]: 98). Along with the relatively modest status accorded to medicine as a profession, the ideas and abilities of physicians significantly to modify the course of illness were not taken to be so very different from those of any well-educated citizen. The lay public could undertake self-treatment and turn to other sources of care. This made sense in the context of the times, when the common belief was that the secrets of medicine were, in fact, limited and very easy to learn. Physicians were thus often seen as dispensable. "Throw by doctors, and be your own Physician, . . . hearkening to them that are used to your Constitution" was the advice given by one well-to-do father to his ill daughter (Karlson and Crumpacker, 1984: 286). The health and healing function was often carried out by someone other than a designated health care provider. That person was more often than not a woman, as women were most likely to stay home and care for the ill. The preacher's wife might consult a handy guide such as Gunn's *Domestic Medicine* (Rosenberg, 1983) or another of the guides that proliferated throughout the country as well as abroad (see Rosenberg, 1983; Lawrence, 1975).

As Rotundo has pointed out, the world of the physician in the nineteenth-century United States shared much with the world of the minister of religion (Rotundo, 1993). Both were of the marketplace, but unlike members of other professions, both spent most of their time dealing with their clients and away from other members of the same profession. In a world of transportation on the back of a horse, absent the now-familiar hospital that draws physicians together, or even the telephone that permits easy communication, the physician and the minister spent much of the day in conversation, often quite casual, with people from all walks of life. And those people tended more often than not to be women. Moreover, members of both professions had as a central part of their mission the duty of caring, of helping family and friends deal with adversity, with counseling and caring when little else was available. In other words, to quote Rotundo, "The essence of each [profession] was nurture" (1993: 208). And nurture often drew representatives of these two professions together. Physicians and the clergy doubtless spent many long hours at the bedside of a sick person, perhaps staying in that same house for days on end, helping to nurse a sick person back to health or to ease the dying person's passage from this world. Caring requires listening, and listening requires time. The nineteenth-century realities of transportation and understandings of disease combined to make it the case that when a physician did arrive at the bedside, she or he was likely to spend considerable time with the patient.

Today, in contrast, physicians spend most of their time talking with each other and not with their patients. Physicians and clergy have grown quite far apart, both in terms of public perceptions and in terms of routinely sharing the same space. In general, the nurturing, caring elements of the medical profession are now less prominent than they were in the nineteenth century. This change may be related to a marked increase in the status of the physician. But before we turn to the transition that has taken place, we should consider in more detail what has already been noted in passing: that during the nineteenth century some women, perceived as having natural caring tendencies, had become physicians.

WOMEN PHYSICIANS: TENSIONS BETWEEN CARING AND SCIENCE

During the second half of the nineteenth century, increasing numbers of women chose to become physicians. The innate characteristics that were believed to make women especially skilled at caregiving followed those women who chose to enter the medical profession, leading to conflict between the need for the new scientific knowledge and the desire to continue in the sympathetic, caring mode (see Morantz-Sanchez, 1985).

The first woman physician to graduate in the United States was Elizabeth Blackwell (1821–1910). She helped to found the women's health movement and was throughout her career an effective and articulate spokesperson for the role of women in medicine and for the need for women to hold onto caring as a part of medicine. Blackwell came of age in an era in which physicians were increasingly turning to the laboratory for insights into health and disease, most prominently in the case of diseases being reconceptualized as caused by small organisms, visible only under a microscope and with special stains. But Blackwell, though well aware of these new currents of medical thought, was not so enamored of the new science. She rejected laboratory medicine in part because it emphasized microbes and tended to draw attention away from the social connectedness of patients. She was also concerned about the increasing practice of vivisection—animal experimentation being done to create new forms of physiological knowledge. She was not so much concerned about the plight of the animals being used for research as she was with the idea that vivisection would contribute to the increased detachment of the physician from the patient—that physicians might come to see their patients as mere "clinical material" rather than as people connected with a family and community (Morantz-Sanchez, 1994, 1999). She was afraid that laboratory medicine would lead physicians to move away from their patients, to treat the body as a machine, and to turn "real patients into objects" (Morantz-Sanchez, 1992: 53). The result would be a medical profession in which caring for the patient would become a less important part of medical practice.

Although Blackwell was hardly alone in questioning the new laboratory medicine—she was joined in her views by many high-profile (usually male) American physicians—what was particularly interesting was the way in which she framed the debate. Blackwell saw physicians as having two duties to their patients. One was to cure disease, to improve functioning—a task that could be enhanced, perhaps, by the new laboratory medicine. But the other task was to relieve suffering through an emotional connection to the patient: she and others of the time would use the word *sympathy*; today, we would call it empathy (Morantz-Sanchez, 1992). Blackwell wanted to use the feminine lessons of maternity to teach "the subordination of the self to the welfare of others; the recognition of the claim which helplessness and ignorance make upon the stronger and more intelligent; the joy of creation and bestowal of life; the pity and sympathy which tend to make every woman the born foe of cruelty and injustice; and hope—which foresees the adult in the infant, the future in the present" (Blackwell, 1902 [1972]: 9–10). Blackwell saw the physician-patient relationship as being modeled on that between mother and child. She carefully pointed out that this sort of interaction could be learned by male physicians as well. Seen in hindsight, her choice of strategies may have hindered their widespread acceptance. Linking her theories with the female sex, a subordinate social group, may not have been the most politically advantageous way to produce change in American medicine. She may have had a better chance of achieving her operational goals had she not based them on theories of feminine difference. Contemporary medicine continues to have similar debates over the extent to which the physician-patient relationship is (or ought to be) defined, and what should be the model of an ideal relationship. The existence of this debate suggests how far caring has fallen from its previous centrality in the physician-patient relationship.

TRANSFORMATION TO THE TWENTIETH CENTURY

The medical transformation of the late nineteenth and the early twentieth centuries transformed not only health care but also caring, with consequences that we live with today.

The Rise of Allopathic Medicine

One important element in this transformation was a revolution in medical education. New ideas, new knowledge, and new technologies made it more difficult for patients to claim to be operating from a similar base of knowledge as the physician. The rise of allopathy led to a new breed of physician—those whom we now recognize through their holding of the M.D. degree. This had important implications for patient care.

Allopathic medicine came to emphasize the natural sciences and to focus on the need to standardize both laboratory observations and the delineation of patient diseases. At the same time, allopathic medicine was often criticized for a perceived lack of caring: healers from other traditions may have been more connected with the community and with the individual characteristics of patients. An example can be seen in the use of X rays and radiation, perhaps the most dramatic of the new medical technologies at the turn of the twentieth century. Whereas allopathic physicians wanted to standardize the use of such rays, homeopathic physicians objected, based on the need to take personal characteristics of the patient into account. One homeopathic commentary asserted, "All these mathematical and physical and chemical methods are dangerous because they do not take into consideration the biological and personal equations. Every roentgenologist of experience knows that the young and old, the sick and well, the anemic and hyperemic, the brunette and blond, the Caucasian and African, react differently" (Dieffenbach, 1923: 712). Perhaps more than allopaths, homeopaths operated within a style of medicine that was attentive to their patients' specific circumstances (Kaufman, 1971). Their approach may account for some of the current popularity of complementary and alternative medicine.

Increased Mobility

Another element in the transformation was a growing number of physicians and the increased ability of doctors to visit patients. Paved roads and the automobile—the latter the subject of a special issue of the *Journal of the American Medical Association* (JAMA) devoted to advising physicians as to whether to buy a car (JAMA, 1912)—combined to make physicians more readily available to see patients in their homes. But simply being able to get to the bedside more easily was not the whole story. Even as physicians became more available, they did not automatically take control of health care. During childbirth, for example, the family did not always defer to the physician's authority. Female relatives of the woman in labor continued to play a central role in decision making: they might decide, for example, whether forceps would be used—and this might be with or without the presence of a physician (Leavitt, 1986). Physicians who cared for patients in their homes for a long period of time often boarded in the house, and this worked against the impression that there was a major status differential between patient and physician. They often had to make do with household equipment or have family assist with procedures (Abel, 1991). The physician's round-the-clock presence also contributed to his or her participation in the day-to-day caring for the patient.

Medical Advances

When a healer had nothing to do but listen to the patient, compassion was part-and-parcel of being a physician. In the early twentieth century, however, new possibilities for action became part of medicine's diagnostic and therapeutic universe. At the same time, these changes had a necessary effect on the ways in which caring and compassion were (or were not) part of the physician's task.

Surgery, for example, was almost miraculous in its new-found ability to invade deep within the body, often with life-saving consequences. Yet, in his marvelous, tightly wound "Indian Camp"—one of the Nick Adams stories—Ernest Hemingway explores how surgery can, and indeed in some instances must, distance the surgeon from the patient (Hemingway, 1972). In this tale, Nick follows his father, a physician, to the "Indian camp" to assist a young, pregnant Native American woman who had been in labor for two days. She is found lying on a lower bunk in a shanty; her husband is on the upper bunk. Nick's father does a cesarean section on the spot and manages to save the mother and child. A cesarean was at the time a rather unusual operation, and afterwards Nick's father is proud of himself. "That's one for the medical journal. . . . Doing a Caesarian with a jackknife and sewing it up with nine-foot, tapered gut leaders." With no anesthetic available, the woman was in considerable pain, but Nick's father says, "Her screams are not important. I don't hear them because they are not important." Perhaps this lack of hearing is understandable. The physician is so intent on doing a technical procedure that he is unable to hear the screams of his patient. Perhaps not hearing the screams enables him to work more effectively, more accurately. In a strictly technical sense, by blocking out the screams he may have been practicing better medicine. But there is clearly a cost to not hearing his patient's pain. In this instance, one cost was the patient's husband (the father of the newborn child). Precisely because, unlike the surgeon, he can hear the screams of his laboring wife, he is found, following the operation, to have quietly cut his own throat "from ear to ear." The new, scientific medicine had enabled (and perhaps required) the physician not to hear the screams of the patient, but her husband had no such respite.

Other scientific advances marked the excitement over turn-of-the-century medicine. The identification of the microorganisms responsible for many human diseases led to the hope that a "magic bullet" could be created to prevent or cure these newly recognized causes of so much human death and disease. Perhaps the ultimate medical miracle of the early years of the century was the discovery of insulin as a treatment for diabetes. Children who had previously been wasting away before the eyes of their grief-stricken parents could be almost instantly transformed into what at first seemed to be the picture of health. The religious implications of this transformation were not lost on contemporary observers. Perhaps a scientific cure was the most appropriate manifestation of caring? But soon the difficulties of long-term insulin treatment were discovered, as diabetes was transformed from an acute into a chronic disease. This general phenomenon—that of a "cure" for an acute disease serving to transform an acute disease into a chronic disease—is one that continued throughout the twentieth century: in the recent past we have the example of the treatment of patients with AIDS. Although the transformation of acute to chronic disease has often been accompanied by discussion of the importance of laboratory science, the results have often increased the need for caring as much as curing.

Another salient feature of the history of early-twentieth-century medicine has been the rise of technology. We have already noted the importance of technology such as the automobile. Other technologies were located in the laboratory, where physicians found that diagnostic clues were to be provided not so much by listening to their patients' voices but by examining their bodily fluids and tissues. The physician was thus drawn away from the bedside and into the laboratory. It should be noted, however, that this was not always the case with new technologies: some, such as the stethoscope, led physicians *to* the bedside, rather than away from it. Other technologies, such as blood counts, could in some cases make a diagnosis that would lead not only to direct physician-patient encounters but also to life-saving operations—surely an example of caring in its finest form (Howell, 1995). On the other hand, overreliance on laboratory values could lead physicians to devote more attention to making the lab values come out right and less to how their patients felt. Patients themselves were afraid that too much reliance on technology would lead physicians to not hear their patients' voices and to lose contact with their patients' wishes.

THE DEVELOPMENT OF INSTITUTIONS AND THE NURSING PROFESSION

Location plays a crucial role in defining how and when caring is done. Prior to the early twentieth century, in a primarily rural society, people who needed care stayed at home. Initially the community would be most important for care, but as families moved increasingly to the frontier, it was the extended family that would care for the person in need. Such a system worked well when families tended to stay close to home. Moreover, with transportation difficult, in many instances there simply was not the option of moving a person who was sick. However, during the early twentieth century, the newly invented institution that came to be known as the modern hospital helped facilitate a separation of seriously ill patients from their communities (Rosenberg, 1987).

The Modern Hospital

The U.S. census of 1920 was the first to show more than 50 percent of the population living in urban areas, then defined as communities with populations greater than two thousand people. With the rise of larger cities, particularly port cities along waterfronts, increasing numbers of young, single men went thither to seek their fortune. They often lived together in apartments. When one person became ill, perhaps as a result of an accident on the busy and dangerous docks, the other people with whom he lived could hardly afford to stay home from work and care for their apartment mate. The injured person thus needed to be cared for in some other place, and the place came to be the hospital. This marked a transition from the earlier role of the hospital, a repository for the dependent poor, toward what we would now call the modern hospital.

The rise of the hospital was also due to a number of other factors. It was a function of the invention of new technologies, both large, bulky, medical ones, such as the X ray and the electrocardiograph machine, and other, business-oriented technologies that made the operation of a large enterprise possible, such as cost accounting and stiff cards called Hollerith cards—a key innovation for manipulating information and the precursor to the IBM punch card that came a few decades later (Howell, 1995). The status of physicians rose along with other professions in the Progressive Era, and hospital care enabled physicians to use their time more efficiently than when they were going from house to house. Surgery became a dominant theme for modern medicine, and efficient operating rooms had much to offer both physician and patient. For these and other reasons, the hospital came to be seen as the appropriate place to go for the care of serious illness. This transition started in the early twentieth century and was essentially completed within a few decades. It was no longer problematic that for the care of acute, life-threatening illness the hospital was the proper place to go, for both rich and poor.

But twentieth-century hospitals did more than take some of the caregiving function away from the local community or the immediate family; they transformed what care was to be like for the acutely ill. When care was given at home, families were intimately involved in all aspects of the patient's care. In early hospitals, in the nineteenth-century, this did not change with the patient's entrance into hospital: families routinely stayed with the ill person, preparing their favorite food and helping to bathe the patient and launder their clothes and bedsheets (a model that still prevails in many hospitals in developing countries). People entered the hospital expecting that they would be able to accompany their relatives everywhere, even into the operating room (Abel, 1991). In the new, modern hospital, that sort of family involvement was no longer desirable or acceptable. The change initially reflected many of the nineteenth-century ideas about the hospital, particularly the sense of moral judgment when hospitals primarily served the destitute. In the earlier era, hospitals kept out visitors in order to establish a strict moral order within the walls

(Vogel, 1980). But twentieth-century hospitals soon found themselves competing for the care of not only the middle-class but also the well-to-do, a group of people who likely did not see themselves as in need of the hospital to impose moral order. For them, the isolation of the patient from outside visitors was based on a different set of assumptions about what would be the best care for the patient. Hospitals argued that they did not want people to be too intimately involved with patients on the grounds that involvement would impede the patient's recovery (Rosner, 1982). Hospitals did offer a place for families of the wealthy to stay in the hospital, but their access to patients was limited. The hospital thus eliminated some of what had constituted the essence of caring.

Hospitalization presented more of an issue for some people than others. At first, hospitals were not universally available, even if desired. Not all people were welcomed in the hospital. African Americans and Native Americans had much less access to hospital care, and for them the burden of care was more likely to remain with the family. In addition, European immigrants were arriving in the United States in increasing numbers. Many of them perceived the country as a land of opportunity. They certainly found opportunity, but they also found considerable prejudice and resentment. Both immigrants and minorities (see Gamble, 1995) feared that when they entered a hospital they would not be well cared for, in every sense of the word. Moreover, due to language difficulties and prejudice, many immigrants found it very hard to get information from hospital staff about their loved ones. There were other reasons they might not wish to enter a hospital. Sometimes the person's work, even when sick, may have been very important for keeping a struggling home afloat.

But at times, immigrants did not want their family members hospitalized because of issues related to caring. While the hospital might be able to treat the organism causing the pneumonia, for example, it simply could not know patients well enough to treat them, to care for them, to provide the sorts of "love and attention they were accustomed to receiving at home" (Abel, 1998: 41)—the sort of caring routinely found in communities before the advent of hospitals.

Family members were attuned to the emotional impact of illness and hospitalization not only in ways that modern, scientific physicians were unaware of but in ways that were positively anathema to the new model of medical care. One woman wrote that her two-year-old son with pneumonia should be released because he "worried so" for his mother; another woman wrote of her husband, "For God sake try and help me to get my husband home he will die of a broken heart be caus he is a way from his family [*sic*]" (Abel, 1998: 43).

Such appeals to compassion were unlikely to be taken seriously by the newly scientific members of the medical profession, increasingly turning to the latest in science and technology as ways to establish themselves as the designated experts for providing health care. The Progressive Era brought increased faith in experts of all types. Authority was to be based on new, technical, verifiable knowledge. For physicians, this new knowledge was based on laboratory medicine, on the definition and characterization of previously undifferentiated disease—a way of knowing that sought standardization and reproducibility above all else (Howell, 1995). In the process, those family members who had been historically most responsible for care—primarily women—lost their authority for caregiving. There was little place here for the knowledge of a patient's temperament, for the sort of intimate, family connection that would be gained by a visit to the person's home. As Abel says, "The new reductionism rendered irrelevant the moral state of the individual, the quality of the interaction between patient and provider, and the nature of a patient's physical surroundings—aspects of healing in which family members had specialized" (Abel, 1991: 53).

The Role of Nursing

The growth of professional nursing, however, enhanced the contact of the healing professions with patients in hospitals as well as in other settings. Around the turn of the twentieth century, there was a marked increase in opportunities for women to pursue a career as a nurse, in part as a function of the same sort of increased urbanization that had led to an increase in the numbers of hospitals. As technological and medical advances increased the amount of information available to physicians, they, in turn, transferred some contact with the reality of their patients' lives to nurses. Nurses increasingly took over the duties of the day-to-day care for patients in hospitals, as well as outside of them. Nurses also helped some families with care in the home, but not all, as many families found that they could not afford the cost (Reverby, 1987).

The caring function that had previously been assumed to some extent by physicians increasingly passed into the world of the nurse. Nurses took over more of the instrumental functions of the physician, the monitoring of blood pressure and pulse, the changing of dressings and the manipulation of injured bodies. Even though in one sense the use of technology such as the sphygmomanometer might lead to a lessening of the caring aspect of medicine, leading as it did to an emphasis on physiological parameters usually not comprehended by the patient, at least the use of instruments to measure blood pressure brought the caregiver into direct contact with the patient, where the nurse could (and usually would) talk to the patient, listen to the patient, and thus have a chance to carry out some basic caring functions. During the post–World War II period, nurses came routinely to use instruments such as stethoscopes and sphygmomanometers at the bedside. Nurses became the ones who comforted people in pain, and the physician became less and less connected with that reality of life and death (Crenner, 1998). At the same time, the physician gained in responsibility and status. Nursing may have gained, too, but it always stayed one step removed from physicians' status. Bad nursing was always a convenient scapegoat for bad outcomes and could be blamed for "thwarting" the best efforts of the physician (Shew, 1882).

Even as nurses acquired new technological skills for patient care, they spent more and more time at the bedside, caring for the emotional needs of their patients, providing empathy as well as medication, both in the hospital as well as in the person's home. Particularly for hospitalized patients, nurses doubtless provided spiritual solace, as well as helping with the practical difficulties of being confined to a hospital. Early in the twentieth century, some hospitals started to employ social workers, who could serve as a bridge to the outside world. They could follow a patient home and ensure that instructions given in the hospital were followed faithfully. In addition, the social worker would try to ensure that the patient's family was well taken care of.

Other Institutions

As hospitals came to be more central for the acute care of the ill, other institutions have come to be seen as more appropriate for long-term care or for care of the dying. The Civil War left large numbers of veterans dependent and in need of caring and led to an interesting early example of a long-term care institution. Perhaps because of the obvious importance of the war for the idea of the United States as a nation, many survivors of it were cared for in large establishments set up specifically for Disabled Volunteer Soldiers, with some of these institutions exceeding five thousand men at their late-nineteenth-century maximum size (Achenbaum, Howell, and Parker, 1993). We can only speculate as to the details of the nature of caring that went on in these homes for disabled soldiers, but the shared Civil War experiences of these veterans may have led to close social relationships among them as they grew old together. Although these nineteenth-century institutions did not survive, wars since that time have often served to redefine patient-caregiver relationships and institutions.

Another type of institution, nursing homes, had their origins in boarding homes and convalescent homes, often sponsored by religious communities. Nursing homes proliferated in the late twentieth century following the enactment of the Medicare and Medicaid programs in 1965. Medicare reimburses posthospital (short-term) care for older and disabled persons; Medicaid reimburses long-term care for chronically ill and disabled persons who meet low-income and asset criteria for eligibility. Nursing homes have become an important component of the health care system.

Hospice is a relatively new system for caring, made necessary in part because hospitals, seemingly focused on curing more than caring, have become less relevant for those who are dying. The first modern hospice was created in 1967 in England near London; the first one in the United States was started in 1974, in New Haven (Sendor and O'Connor, 1997), and Medicare began funding hospice care in 1982. Interesting differences between the hospice movements in the two countries highlight the importance of social context. In England, the medical model takes a comparatively broad and encompassing view of a wide range of human needs. English hospice programs were begun with physicians as leaders; founded by Cicely Saunders (later to be Dame Cicely Saunders), from the start they were both intellectually and operationally part of the medical community and the National Health Service. In the United States, the programs were created out of a belief that the medical system was itself failing the caring needs of the dying, and thus hospice programs often were separated from the medical establishment, although the medical system has recently come to interact much more closely with hospices. Medical care in hospices is provided by physicians and nurses, much as in hospitals, but substantial caring in these programs is provided by social workers, chaplains, and volunteers.

Hospice is increasingly being seen as central to the medical mission. In 1997, it was reported that 17 percent of those who die receive hospice care (Field and Cassel, 1997); this care is primarily provided in the homes of patients (Moore and McCollough, 2000). Nonetheless, the elderly and seriously ill are now far more often likely to die in hospitals and other institutions than in the past, when they were cared for and died in their homes or in the homes of their families. According to an Institute of Medicine report (Field and Cassel, 1997), in 1949 about 50 percent of Americans died in hospitals and other institutions; by 1992, 57 percent of deaths occurred in hospitals, 17 percent in nursing homes, 20 percent in residences, and 6 percent elsewhere (including those declared dead on arrival at the hospital).

There were relatively few paid professionals involved in home health care prior to the mid-1980s. However, following a 1989 liberalization of federal eligibility criteria for home health care services reimbursed by Medicare (as the result of a lawsuit), there was a tremendous growth in the volume of such services and persons who used them. From 1988 through 1996, the number of home health visits per thousand Medicare enrollees grew by 587 percent, and the number of persons served increased 125 percent. As a consequence, during this period Medicare payments to home health agencies increased by 762 percent, from $1.9 billion to $16.8 billion (Binstock and Cluff, 2000). By 1996, the total national expenditure for home care providers, from all sources, had reached $31.2 billion, with 91 percent of it funded by Medicare and Medicaid, including expenditures for hospice home care (Levit et al., 1998). Although total spending increased dramatically, it is unclear what benefit (if any) has resulted from it or whether those with greatest need have been the recipients of such services.

Institutions for the mentally ill once played a major role in caring for people with many types of mental difficulty, including elderly persons thought to have "dementia." During the deinstitutionalization movement of the 1960s large numbers of people moved out of institutions designed to care for the mentally ill. The percentage of elderly people in such institutions dropped from 23 percent in 1950 to 10 percent in 1970 (Kane, Kane, and Ladd, 1998); many of them are now cared for in different settings such as "halfway houses" or, often, in the homes of their families. Many others who were deinstitutionalized have become self-sufficient with the aid of medication. And still others are homeless.

BACK TO THE FUTURE?

The trend to move people out of hospitalized care sooner, to have them go back to home and community and family, is superficially reminiscent of the nineteenth-century world we visited earlier. There are indeed similarities, but there are important differences as well. Today, as then, families take on most of the responsibility for caregiving. But families are now more dispersed than they were in the past. As families moved farther and farther into the new frontier, as several generations of a family were less and less likely to stay in the same place, the responsibility for caring became diffused and attenuated. Improved communication has made possible the occasional telephone call, and improved transportation has certainly enabled families to return more easily (and perhaps more often) to visit their loved ones, by train, car, and plane. But there is a huge difference between periodically visiting a loved one and living in the same neighborhood or household. Perhaps as a result of families moving farther apart, perhaps as a consequence of the increasing urbanization of society, loneliness has become practically epidemic in American society. Whereas caring for one's neighbors was once a widely accepted communal responsibility, now people feel that merely calling on a neighbor can be an imposition (Gordon, 1976). There is not the same sort of generally accepted responsibility within a close-knit community as was the case in the nineteenth century.

In our more organized world, public policy does not reflect or support the centrality of families in caring for those in need (Levine, 1999). Today's families are likely to incur heavy costs in ensuring care for a family member, both in direct costs and in the burden of lost wages and lost time spent caring for others. And within families, who is doing the caring? Since at least the middle of the nineteenth century, women have been assumed to be the most natural providers of care, a gender-based division that persists. As before, the burden has tended to fall disproportionately on women (Brody, 1990).

But radically new changes have taken place over recent decades. Two new features have come to dominate the health care scene, both of which have significant implications for caring. One is the recent availability of information-management technology. Derived from the Hollerith cards of the early twentieth century, these new information technologies enable data management of a previously unimaginable scale and scope. Combined with the move toward integrated delivery systems for defined groups of patients, they raise the possibility of effective population-based health care. By tracking and encouraging the use of interventions and technologies that have been shown to both prolong life and improve the quality of life, we may be able to care much more effectively for groups of patients. Physicians can now be judged on the basis of how well they are caring for a panel of patients, as well as for individual patients. We could choose to use that information to measure and encourage medicine aimed at doing the most good for the greatest number, to reconnect with the community, albeit in a different way.

The second major change has been the rise of patient autonomy as an omnipresent mantra for all health care decisions. Perhaps autonomy has long been established in a personal sense, but in a medical sense this transition is quite recent. It is easy to forget how recently leading scholars, legislators, and policymakers debated autonomy in the medical setting, as exemplified in the title of a book from the 1950s, *Should the Patient Know the Truth?* (Standard and Nathan, 1955). Now there is little doubt that competent patients are entitled, as a matter of ethics and law, to any and all information about their health care that they wish to have. This truly revolutionary change in the approach to health care means that in the future we may wish to speak of caring "with" as much as "for" the patient. In so doing, we may give voice to the multiple and varying priorities that our patients hold, and in so doing become even more effective at truly caring for those in need.

Both of these changes have had a major impact on the role of physicians, who have come to dominate medical practice in the United States. Early in the twentieth century, physicians started out with a broad model of caring for the patient. The model of patient care then became narrower, partly as a result of economics, partly as a result of specialization, partly as a result of technology. In addition to technological and medical advances, the relative economic status of physicians has improved, resulting in physicians no longer being as well connected as before to the communities that they serve. Today's physicians are more likely to be found at the country club than at the bowling alley. Another characteristic of twentieth-century medical practice is the increasing specialization of physicians. Specialists and hospitalists are likely to "see" a critically ill patient first as an X ray or a CAT scan, and then to meet that patient in person for the first time when he or she is in a hospital bed, garbed in a hospital gown and disconnected from most traces of the patient's life outside of the institution. It is thus not a surprise that there is little (or no) preexisting social connection on which the physician-patient relationship can rest. Although the rhetoric of caring is generally espoused, in many fields such rhetoric is too often subsumed beneath an overlay of science and technology.

Yet, as we begin the twenty-first century, there are signs that the importance of caring in medical care will be enhanced. There are fields of medicine that tend to spend more time addressing issues of caring, such as internal medicine, family medicine, pediatrics, and geriatrics. Although these specialties tend, by and large, to be less-well-paid than the more technologically intensive specialties, these patient-centered fields have recently begun to attract more attention, perhaps as a result of societal attitudes about primary care, about "patient-centered care" (Brown, 1986). It is also possible that new types of technology that enable physicians to measure and be measured in terms of a broader model of what they do for populations of patients will also increase the extent to which physicians reassume the role of caring for their patients as well as tending to their medical needs.

ACKNOWLEDGMENTS

The author greatly appreciates insightful suggestions and comments from Emily Abel, Tracy Crew, Kenneth Langa, Regina Morantz-Sanchez, Andrea Sankar, and the Division of General Medicine at the University of Michigan. Preparation of this chapter was supported by an Investigator Award in Health Policy Research from the Robert Wood Johnson Foundation and by a Burroughs Wellcome Fund Tenth Anniversary Award in the History of Medicine and Science.

REFERENCES

Abel, E. K. (1991). *Who Cares for the Elderly? Public Policy and the Experiences of Adult Daughters.* Philadelphia, PA: Temple University Press.

Abel, E. K. (1998). Turn-of-the-century conflicts between charity workers and women clients. *Journal of Woman's History* 10: 32–52.

Abel, E. K. (2000). *Hearts of Wisdom: American Women Caring for Kin, 1850–1940.* Cambridge: Harvard University Press.

Achenbaum, A., Howell, J. D., and Parker, M. (1993). Patterns of alcohol use and abuse among aging Civil War veterans, 1865–1920. *Bulletin of the New York Academy of Medicine* 69: 69–85.

Baker, P. (1984). The domestication of politics: Women and American political society, 1780–1920. *American Historical Review* 89: 620–47.

Binstock, R. H., and Cluff, L. E. (2000). Issues and challenges in home care. In R. H. Binstock and L. W. Cluff, eds., *Home Care Advances: Essential Research and Policy Issues,* pp. 3–34. New York: Springer Publishing.

Blackwell, E. (1902 [1972]). The influence of women in the profession of medicine. In *Essays in Medical Sociology.* Reprint, New York: Arno Press. Quoted in Morantz-Sanchez, 1994.

Brody, E. M. (1990). *Women in the Middle: Their Parent-Care Years.* New York: Springer Publishing.

Brown, T. M. (1986). American medicine and primary care: The last half-century.

In S. J. Kunitz, ed., *The Training of Primary Physicians*, pp. 1–58. Lanham, MD: University Press of America.

Cathell, D. W. (1890). *Book on the Physician Himself and Things that Concern His Reputation and Success.* 9th ed. Philadelphia, PA: F. A. Davis.

Crenner, C. (1998). Introduction of the blood pressure cuff into U.S. medical practice: Technology and skilled practice. *Annals of Internal Medicine* 126: 488–93.

Demos, J. (1970). *A Little Commonwealth: Family Life in Plymouth Colony.* New York: Oxford University Press.

Dieffenbach, W. H. (1923). A brief historical review and the present status of roentgenotherapy. *Hahnemannian Monthly* 58: 711–20.

Farrar, E. W. (1837). *The Young Lady's Friend—by a Lady.* Boston, MA: American Stationer's. Quoted in S. Reverby, 1990. The duty or right to care? Nursing and womanhood in historical perspective. In E. K. Abel and M. K. Nelson, eds., *Circles of Care: Work and Identity in Women's Lives*, pp. 132–49. Albany: State University of New York.

Field, M. J., and Cassel, C. K. (1997). *Approaching Death: Improving Care at the End of Life.* Washington, DC: National Academy Press.

Gamble, V. (1995). *Making a Place for Ourselves: The Black Hospital Movement, 1920–1945.* New York: Oxford University Press.

Gordon, S. (1976). *Lonely in America.* New York: Simon & Schuster.

Gunn, J. (1830 [1986]). *Gunn's Domestic Medicine, or Poor Man's Friend.* Printed under the immediate superintendance [*sic*] of the author, a physician of Knoxville; reprint, 1986, Knoxville: University of Tennessee Press.

Hemingway, E. (1972). Indian camp. In *The Nick Adams Stories*, pp. 16–21. New York: Charles Scribner's Sons.

Howell, J. D. (1995). *Technology in the Hospital: Transforming Patient Care in the Early Twentieth Century.* Baltimore: Johns Hopkins University Press.

Howell, J. D. (1997). Making medical practice in an uneasy world: Some thoughts from a century ago. *Academic Medicine* 72: 977–81.

Journal of the American Medical Association (1912). Satisfaction in automobiling: A symposium by physicians on their experience with motor-cars—How to secure the most in comfort and help at the least expense. 58: 1049–70.

Kane, R. A., Kane, R. L., and Ladd, R. C. (1998). *The Heart of Long-Term Care.* New York: Oxford University Press.

Karlson, C. F., and Crumpacker, L., eds. (1984). *The Journal of Esther Edwards Burr, 1754–1757.* New Haven: Yale University Press.

Kaufman, M. (1971). *Homeopathy in America: The Rise and Fall of a Medical Heresy.* Baltimore: Johns Hopkins University Press.

Lawrence, C. J. (1975). William Buchanan: Medicine laid open. *Medical History* 19: 20–35.

Leavitt, J. (1986). *Brought to Bed: Child-Bearing in America, 1750–1950.* New York: Oxford University Press.

Levine, C. (1999). The loneliness of the long-term care giver. *New England Journal of Medicine* 340: 1587–90.

Levit, K., Cowan, C., Braden, B., Stiller, J., Sensenig, A., and Lazenby, H. (1998). National health expenditures in 1997: More slow growth. *Health Affairs* 17(6): 99–110.

Moore, P. C., and McCollough, R. H. (2000). Hospice: End-of-life care. In R. H. Binstock and L. E. Cluff, eds., *Home Care Advances: Essential Research and Policy Issues,* pp. 101–16. New York: Springer Publishing.

Morantz-Sanchez, R. (1985). *Sympathy and Science: Women Physicians in American Medicine.* New York: Oxford University Press.

Morantz-Sanchez, R. (1992). Feminist theory and historical practice: Rereading Elizabeth Blackwell. *History and Theory* 31: 31–69.

Morantz-Sanchez, R. (1994). The gendering of empathic expertise: How women physicians became more empathic than men. In E. S. More and M. A. Milligan, eds., *The Empathic Practitioner: Empathy, Gender, and Medicine,* pp. 40–58. New Brunswick, NJ: Rutgers University Press.

Morantz-Sanchez, R. (1999). *Conduct Unbecoming a Woman: Medicine on Trial in Turn-of-the-Century Brooklyn.* New York: Oxford University Press.

Murphy, L. M. (1991). *Enter the Physician: The Transformation of Domestic Medicine 1760–1860.* Tuscaloosa: University of Alabama Press.

Nightingale, F. (1860 [1969]). *Notes on Nursing: What It Is and What It Is Not.* New York: Appleton; reprint, New York: Dover.

Reverby, S. (1987). *Ordered to Care: The Dilemma of American Nursing, 1850–1945.* Cambridge: Cambridge University Press.

Rosenberg, C. E. (1979). The therapeutic revolution. In M. J. Vogel and C. E. Rosenberg, eds., *The Therapeutic Revolution: Essays in the Social History of American Medicine,* pp. 3–25. Philadelphia: University of Pennsylvania Press.

Rosenberg, C. E. (1983). Medical text and social context: Explaining William Buchanan's *Domestic Medicine. Bulletin of the History of Medicine* 57: 22–42.

Rosenberg, C. E. (1986). John Gunn, everyman's physician. Introduction to *Gunn's Domestic Medicine, or, Poor Man's Friend.* A facsimile of the first edition: With an introduction by Charles E. Rosenberg. Knoxville: University of Tennessee Press.

Rosenberg, C. E. (1987). *The Care of Strangers: The Rise of America's Hospital System.* New York: Basic Books.

Rosner, D. (1982). *A Once Charitable Enterprise: Hospitals and Health Care in Brooklyn and New York, 1885–1915.* Cambridge: Cambridge University Press.

Rotundo, E. A. (1993). *American Manhood: Transformations in Masculinity from the Revolution to the Modern Era.* New York: Basic Books.

Sendor, V. F., and O'Connor, P. M. (1997). *Hospice and Palliative Care.* Lanham, MD: Scarecrow Press.

Shew, J. (1882). *The Hydropathic Family Physician.* New York: Fowler & Wells.

Standard, S., and Nathan, H. (1955). *Should the Patient Know the Truth?* New York: Springer Publishing.

Vogel, M. (1980). *The Invention of the Modern Hospital: Boston, 1870–1930.* Chicago: University of Chicago Press.

5

Forces Affecting Caring by Physicians

ERIC J. CASSELL, M.D.

IT WOULD BE simple to point to surface factors that keep physicians from being more fully engaged in caring, such as the values conveyed through graduate medical education or methods of reimbursement for medical care. There is no question that changes in these areas and others would bring medicine closer to being a caring profession. I do not believe, however, that calling for such revisions will be sufficient without recognition of the profoundly influential intellectual and cultural forces that reduced the importance of caring in contemporary medicine. Why? Because bringing about change against a strong and deep current requires different actions than even persuasive arguments and excellent suggestions in a world ready to listen. Here, not only is the goal worth the effort for medicine, but medicine is very influential in bringing about needed equivalent changes in society even while it is society's child. So let me spend some time on the pathogenesis of medicine's illness, the apparent loss of the ability and the desire to care.

WHERE IS CARING IN THE HISTORIES OF MEDICINE?

It is frequently said that until the 1920s or 1930s there was nothing definitive that a physician could do for a sick person. At first hearing this seems odd because no system of medicine survives unless it is effective, and Hippocratic medicine has been in existence for more than 2,400 years, fundamentally unchanged. We know from history that some doctors were more effective than others, but what they actually did to help their patients seems closed to us. We are so rooted in the present era of effective therapeutics that we can only presume that earlier physicians in the Hippocratic tradition made their patients better through their actions as caregivers and healers—although what that actually meant in practice I do not know. Of course, patient expectations were derivative from their knowledge of what was possible, and thus quite different from what patients currently expect.

For several hundred years, most attention has been paid to the empirical method of Hippocratic medicine—the close observation and description of the sick—as a basis for physicians' actions. This first appeared in the Hippocratic writings, was revived by Thomas Sydenham and then John Locke in the seventeenth century (Albutt, 1911; Coulter, 1988; King, 1978), and ultimately paved the way for the entrance of modern science into medicine. For the most part, standard histories of medicine, rather than focusing on what physicians actually did, concentrate on the steady accretion of knowledge of the body and the nature of disease, particularly since the sixteenth century. This is the way we tend to think about medicine; to have knowledge of the workings of the body in disease is to have mastery over disease. To know science is to know medicine. This understanding of medicine slipped so naturally into the current era that we do not concentrate on the radical discontinuity of the content of medical practice between the past and now.

If this brief recital stopped here, then it would be possible to proceed to a demonstration of the current impedimenta to caring and their solution with an innocent belief in the efficacy of the prescription. Unfortunately, there are sets of fundamental ideas about science and technology that increasingly cause physicians to neglect caring for their patients while focusing on their disease states or bodily malfunctions. These ideas have power, in part because physicians are unaware of them in their thoughts and actions and in part because they pervade not only medicine but also the whole culture. They all derive from the centrality of science in medicine and also in much of Western society, a pride of place that existed for most of the twentieth century. Because Western schoolchildren are steeped in science and scientific assumptions from their earliest days, these beliefs are as much a part of the thinking of contemporary physicians as the idea of God was three hundred years ago.

THE GOALS AND CHALLENGES OF CARING

In Daniel Callahan's wonderful contribution to this volume (see chapter 1) he tells us that caring is needed to maximize function, help patients recover their autonomy, relieve pain and suffering, provide physical and psychological security in the midst of the deprivations and uncertainties of illness, and recognize patients' psychological and spiritual needs. He makes clear that meeting these goals requires recognizing and responding to patients' cognitive needs for knowledge and information, meeting specific emotional needs, accomplishing these goals in terms of the particular patient's values—what is important to *this* patient—and facilitating the patient's relationships and interactions with others.

In order to do these things, doctors must be more than personally caring or compassionate. They must have the skill to bring their scientific and technical knowledge of medicine to bear on the needs, desires, concerns, fears, hopes, and purposes of *this* patient as they arise and evolve in the course of the illness, whatever its outcome. They must integrate facts, from both the body and the many dimensions of the person, with the theoretical knowledge and perspective developed in their training and maintained in Western medicine's worldview.

Because caring is concerned with the welfare of others, it is primarily a *moral* endeavor, taking place in the domain of what is right and good. But when it is medical caring, it also requires the technical for its performance. The technical requirements of medical caring should disabuse us of the belief that the caring that physicians do in their families—a natural behavior common to many—need only be brought over into their professional work. This is not the case. The way people act in the public and professional world may be greatly different than their private and personal behavior. The former is guided by one set of rules and the latter by a different set of norms. It is the systematic scheme of ideas that underlie the thoughts and actions of physicians in their professional lives with which we are concerned.

KEY CONCEPTS THAT UNDERLIE SCIENCE AND MEDICINE

Three key trends concern us here. The first is the rise of the worldview of science, often associated with the words *positivism, logical positivism, scientific materialism,* and *logical empiricism.* In this worldview, the only valid information comes from science, which deals only in experiential and verifiable facts. Facts, in this perspective, are atomistic; they are separate from other facts and are individually verifiable. They are not necessarily connected in a way such that all facts are believed to be related to each other and part of a system embedded in a way of seeing and understanding the world. Such systems, in this view, are metaphysical, only speculative, and of no value. Any statements that cannot actually or potentially be factually verified are meaningless (so the beliefs go) or, like statements in the realm of values or the moral, are at best matters of opinion or taste. Facts that meet the ideal are obtained by reducing wholes to their most basic parts in such a manner that the observation of the parts can be rigorously controlled. Knowledge of the whole is gained, in this view, by knowledge of the parts.

The second trend is the common medical belief that only that which is objective provides useful information. Subjective information arising from values, feelings, opinions, or beliefs is thought to be flawed, unreliable, and, in scientific terms, meaningless. In this way, the subject that is the patient (and the subject that is the physician) is disvalued relative to the object that is the body (or its parts), disease, or pathophysiology. Physicians can relate to this last because the dominance of this idea (the denigration of the subjective) is everywhere in medicine—in undergraduate and graduate medical education, in journals, and in the day-to-day language of teachers and practitioners. Ideas about objective versus subjective information are clearly related to the embrace of the scientific worldview.

The third and related trend separates human beings from the remainder of nature (including their bodies) because nature is seen to be an entirely material world of random forces divorced from any ideas of purposeful behavior that are associated with humankind. This modern duality has been included as one of the modern meanings of nihilism: the world has no meaning; in fact, nothing except humans has meaning or purpose. There are no overriding or transcendent purposes. The effect of these ideas is to create a subject-object duality. In the words of Robert Pirsig in *Zen and the Art of Motorcycle Maintenance:*

> For true science to take place these [subject and object] must be rigidly separate from each other. "You are the mechanic. There is the motorcycle. You are forever apart from one another. You do this to it. You do that to it. These will be the results."
>
> This eternally dualistic subject-object way of approaching the motorcycle sounds right to us because we're used to it. But it's not right. It's always been an artificial interpretation *superimposed* on reality. It's never been reality itself. When this duality is completely accepted a certain

> non-divided relationship between the mechanic and the motorcycle, a craftsmanlike feeling for the work is destroyed. When traditional rationality divides the world into subjects and objects it shuts out Quality, and when you're really stuck it's Quality . . . that tells you where you ought to go. (Pirsig, 1979: 282)

It is not difficult to see the obstacles that these trends put in the way of caring for patients, their families, and their communities by physicians in whom these beliefs occupy a dominant, although mostly invisible, place. Unfortunately, conceptual difficulties do not stop here. Hippocratic medicine gave Western medicine not only its scientific spirit but also its ethical ideals. Until recent generations, the guiding ethical principles of medicine have been benevolence and the avoidance of harm. In the words of Bela Schick, "First the patient, second the patient, third the patient, fourth the patient, fifth the patient, and then maybe comes science" (Wilkins, 1991: 11). For ages, the centrality of the patient has been much spoken about, although in recent times the words have been empty.

BIOETHICS AND THE SOCIAL CLIMATE OF MEDICINE

Since the 1950s, during the same period in which science achieved its virtually complete dominance as a route to knowledge, the bioethics movement has also achieved great influence in medicine (see Rothman, 1991). As a consequence, the idea that the *primary* ethical motivation of physicians should be to do good for their patients and avoid harm began to give way. Benevolence in action often entailed physicians' ideas of what was good and what was harmful. In cultures in which personal aspirations and values were believed to be relatively uniform (e.g., in the United States before World War II), it seemed reasonable that physicians' knowledge of what was good and right for the sick would serve as a reliable guide to benevolent actions. The custom of physicians acting independently for their patients was reinforced by the widespread social acceptance of their authority, coupled with the well-intentioned practice of concealing the truth from patients, which prevented their meaningful participation in decisions about their own care.

The social climate of the United States during the 1960s—the period that saw the origins of contemporary bioethics—was marked by changes that had a profound impact on medical practice. The civil-rights movement, focusing initially on blacks in the South, spread across the country and then found expression in the women's movement, the gay-rights movement, the rights movement of persons with disabilities, and ultimately spread to patients ("treat the patient as a person"). The social ideal of commonality in American values gave way to pride in diversity. An increasing individualism emphasized the importance of persons and their rights and choices. All authority, including that of physicians, came into question. The bioethics movement, arriving on the scene in the late 1960s and early 1970s, pronounced traditional physician benevolence a form of paternalism that ill-fitted the new central concept of respect for persons (Beauchamp and Childress, 1994; Childress, 1982).

Patient autonomy became the highest value (Schneider, 1998). In action, this demanded of physicians that they respect and enhance freedom of choice by patients. This required new standards for the disclosure of information, truth telling, and patient participation in decision making. Now patients could not only be harmed by physicians, a failure of the ideal of benevolence, they could be wronged, a moral and legal notion. The image of the autonomous patient began to approximate the idea of persons common in the law—separate and atomistic. In this worldview, it was no longer the physician operating through a special relationship that was crucial to the treatment of patients, it was science and technology that did the work. At the same time, ideas of the importance and centrality of the relationship between patient and physician diminished and assumed a nostalgic quality.

Further, the actions of physicians began to be "commodified." As examples, an office visit for a minor illness, a physical examination, reading an electrocardiogram, a digital rectal examination—previously merely things that were done as part of taking care of patients—now became billable medical commodities. As commodities and thus part of the resources of the health care system, their meaning shifted. They were no longer solely part of the interaction of patient and physician—medical exemplifications of benevolence. Now they and their allocation could be examined through the lens of equity and justice. Thus a physician who did not adequately relieve a patient's pain was not merely failing to care for the patient, breaching the duty of benevolence, but was acting unjustly by withholding pain-relieving resources.

Justice and benevolence are in two different moral worlds. The failure of benevolence is failure of a professional moral duty, whereas being unjust is in the moral universe of the law and politics. Its recognition as applicable to medicine denies the importance of the moral bond between patient and physician.

CHANGING NOTIONS OF BENEVOLENCE

The medical ideal of benevolence—to do good for the *patient* and avoid harm to the *patient*—has itself changed within the last generation, further moving physicians from caring for patients. We were not far into the era of modern definitions of disease—say, the middle or end of the nineteenth century—when doing good for the patient was clearly equated with doing good for the disease. As Sir William Gull (1816–90) was moved to say, "Never forget that it is not a pneumonia, but a pneumonic man who is your patient" (Wilkins, 1991: 11). The difficulties of having physicians maintain responsibility for the whole patient increased, however, with the growing effectiveness of medical interventions and need for specialists and special services.

In the care of the dying, the paradoxes of benevolence are easily seen. The goal of keeping people alive entered medicine in the nineteenth century, well before the necessary technical capability existed. By the third quarter of the twentieth century, however, resuscitation techniques and life-extending therapies made it possible to keep patients alive who would previously have died of their diseases. Even patients in the terminal stages of their disease (e.g., cancer, emphysema, massive stroke) and surely soon to die could be maintained alive for a while longer by advanced life-support systems. It came to be believed, as reflected in law and regulations, that remaining alive was the ultimate good, whatever the future might hold. On this basis, the judgment of physicians about which patients should be resuscitated was superceded by legal requirements that resuscitation be attempted for all patients whatever their cause of death. Only a directive to the contrary signed by the patient when competent could be the basis of a legal "do not resuscitate" order.

By the 1980s, intensive care units in hospitals contained patients on life support even when they had no chance of return to meaningful life whatever the outcome of life-support therapies. The floors of hospitals contained bed after bed in which some old woman (fewer men survived long enough to reach this state) with advanced, progressive, irremediable Alzheimer disease or other dementia was maintained alive by the treatment of one infectious or metabolic complication after another. Here again, law mandated continued treatment unless the patient had a legal advance directive to the contrary or a legal surrogate. Because of fears of malpractice or other legal action, such treatment was given in the absence of specific laws requiring it even if physicians believed such therapy not to be in the best interests of the patient. The implication of these laws, regulations, and fears of legal action was to redefine medical beneficence in technical terms, and keeping someone alive "at all costs" became a medical good.

Medical advances increasingly made it possible to support individual physiological functions independently of the state of the whole patient. Renal dialysis, ever-better ventilators, pacemakers and many other cardiac-support techniques, various modes of blood-pressure support, total parenteral nutrition, transfusion of blood components, various bone marrow stimulants to resolve anemia, leukopenia, and thrombocytopenia, and others all permitted the treatment of failing organ, biochemical, and physiological systems, whether or not such therapy met a larger definition of good for the sick person. I have described primarily medical therapies, but the point could be made as well with surgical techniques.

THE ROMANCE OF ACUTE ILLNESS (AND THE NEGLECT OF THE CHRONIC)

The therapeutic advances I have described primarily focus on acute events. Consequently, chronic illnesses such as diabetes, coronary heart disease, stroke, cancer, AIDS, and neurological disorders are often treated as a series of acute episodes. From this perspective, it is possible to consider the abnormal process completely apart from the person in whom it occurs. The technical details of ventilator support in lung failure are independent of the particular patient. Some patients tolerate the treatment better and some worse. Some are more frightened and are less cooperative, and others are more or less demanding. These are the personal characteristics of the patients. They can be seen as (say) helpful or annoying in terms of the dominant technical task but not an inherent part of the clinical situation that requires caring.

Medicine that is primarily concerned with acute events continues to define the major focus of clinical policy—the aggregate of medical education, hospital care, medical insurance, ambulatory services, medical research, and all the other facets of the institution of medicine—including, as we have seen, definitions of benevolence. Yet, focusing on the acute distorts reality. Since the 1920s and progressively so in the decades after World War II, the chronic diseases have been the major cause of mortality and morbidity. They consume the most medical care, and particularly in an aging population they are overwhelmingly the most common causes of the impairments that demand caring if the needs of the patient are to be adequately met (Kramer, 1996).

CARING IS OUTSIDE THE PALE—RECAP OF FUNDAMENTAL REASONS

It is a delusion to believe that the nature of the sick person and the importance of caring are not central in the care of patients with acute events. One would think it impossible to hold the delusion in relation to chronic disease. Not so. Caring, unfortunately, is simply defined as outside the realm of mainstream medicine. This should hardly be surprising.

To recapitulate, medical thinking is ruled by the worldview of twentieth-century biological science, which values atomistic verifiable facts and disvalues the moral, and values. Further, the objective and objectivity rank much higher than the subjective and subjectivity. Finally, these ideas and others that guide biological science's view of nature (including humankind) have created a subject-object duality that further separates humans from their own bodies. As a social reflection of these concepts, the increasing individuality that marks persons in the United States is mirrored in bioethics by an emphasis on the autonomous patient, whose characteristics are similar to the narrow and atomistic definition of a person as seen in the law. Indeed, the major moral force in medicine since antiquity, benevolence, has been moved aside by the emphasis on autonomy. To be sure, benevolence and a fear of harming patients (which lives inside clinicians all of their working lives) remain important moral forces, despite the decrease in importance of the doctor-patient relationship to the institutions of medicine. The form of benevolence, however, has changed progressively over the past several decades. It now seems less concerned with the whole person and increasingly focused on the person's parts and pathophysiology. Once almost exclusively the domain of the clinician, the definition of what counts for the good of the patient is increasingly the province of the patient (independent of the physician), the law, and the third-party payer.

THE IMPACT OF TECHNOLOGY

The role of technology in defeating caring cannot be overestimated. The growth of technology is probably the primary factor in the escalating cost of medical care in the United States and other developed countries.

Its grip on medical practice and physician behavior is so tight that it has squeezed out the personal diagnostic and therapeutic skills of physicians. It has been repeatedly documented, for example, that the quality of the basic clinical skills of physicians—specifically, the ability to take histories from patients and do physical examinations—has diminished in recent years as reliance on diagnostic technology and therapeutic technology has increased (Bardes, 1998). I do not mean merely simpler things like stethoscopes and reflex hammers that make it possible for physicians to hear better or see better, yet still fundamentally rely on their senses and judgment. These devices do not divert the purposes of their users to the purposes of the technology. Rather, I am talking about diagnostic and therapeutic modalities that extend the *power* of the physician many times over, as exemplified by the MRI, CT, antibiotics, psychotropic drugs, and so forth, that cause themselves to be employed as though they had a life of their own. The hold of advanced technology on medicine is something like the sorcerer's broom in the fairy tale—what started off under the control of physicians has now assumed an unstoppable life of its own (see Cassell, 1993).

Technologies are reductive and oversimplifying. Much of their hold on physicians is a result of two prior reductive steps in the history of medicine. The first was reducing the complex and multifaceted problem of human illness to the biological problem of disease. The second reductive step resulting from the scientific investigation of disease was that the findings of science became the accepted picture of disease, further oversimplifying the matter; the picture excluded, for example, personal or social dimensions. The technology is generated from the scientific understanding and, itself, further confirms the scientific picture.

Technology commands as it does because of certain human traits that seem to make it beckon more vigorously than any patient's unmet need for caring. There are five characteristics of technology that require attention if it is to be brought back under control.

The first is the wonder and fascination induced by anything new that does fantastic or apparently inexplicable things. This motivation for the use of technology is present throughout the society and recognizable at all ages. In medicine, it causes people to use their technology when clearly indicated, but also to extend its use inappropriately just for the pleasure of it.

The second characteristic is the lure of the immediate. The numbers on the readout, the image on the film, technical dexterity required for deployment, the details of the equipment—all these exist in the here and now, the immediate moment. Technology's output is immediate in another important sense; it is unmediated by human reason. What you see is what you get. The result speaks for itself. It is not unusual for physicians to accept the result of an MRI, for example—what they believe they see on the films—when the result is anatomically or physiologically impossible. The image displaces reason. How different are patients and their need for caring! If you look at patients and see only the immediate here and now, you will miss what is important. Given the complexity and the difficulty in understanding patients, the lure of the immediacy of advanced technology is not surprising.

The third reason for technology's hold on physicians is the lure of the unambiguous. Criteria developed for technologies are usually very clear. We have come to know what a good coronary angiogram looks like, and how a "good" coronary artery differs from a "bad" one on the films. This year's films can be compared with the previous study using clear criteria for difference. Similarly, the numbers on an automated chemistry printout fit criteria for normalcy or otherwise. Physicians come to accept these apparently unambiguous results as though nature was similarly unambiguous. Emphatically, it is not. But patients are made to worry about abnormalities in blood-chemistry results that, although above the line of normal, are of no clinical importance. Physicians' acceptance of the numbers has apparently pushed their knowledge of the body to the side. Very little in human experience of any importance is similarly unambiguous. In fact, with sophistication in any area comes appreciation of ambiguities.

The fourth, and perhaps the most important feature of technology that helps explain its hold on medicine, is its ability to reduce uncertainty. Central to learning to be a clinician is learning to accept uncertainty as inevitable and learning strategies to reduce its toll. Technologies—CT, MRI, endoscopies, cardiac electrophysiology, chemistries, and on and on—appear to remove uncertainty. The days of wondering what was in the abdomen before a laporotomy, or whether more or less digitalis glycoside should be given; of waiting for the next episode (or episodes) for the disease to reveal itself—these days are over in many areas of medicine. Good riddance! Often, however, the certainty is achieved by converting a complex problem into a simple one. For example, transforming the difficult problem of back pain to the results of an MRI of the spine may seem to be a reasonable way to proceed. But MRIs of the spine may show up as "abnormal" when pain is absent or "normal" when it is present. And rarely do they reveal why the patient has back pain. Or consider a case in which, for instance, a sick person's illness is converted into the problems of an organ so that episodes of chest pain or other symptoms are interpreted as possibly being cardiac. If the tests are negative, the patient is told that he does not have heart disease. Even if true, the original question was not whether heart disease was present, but why the patient is symptomatic.

After a decade of saturation with technology, one of the most distressing results has been a whole cohort of physicians unable to manage their or their patients' uncertainties. Uncertainty, unfortunately, never disappears. It is the inevitable accompaniment of the fact that all medical care takes place in and has its impact on the future (starting a moment from now), that knowledge is never complete, and that the knowledge of medical science is about universals. But all patients are unique and particular. There are so many uncertainties about the proper form of caring that doctors who cannot tolerate uncertainty may be forced away from it by their inability to manage it.

The fifth reason that caring is impeded by unmanaged technological growth is that technology is self-perpetuating. The proliferation of technology in intensive care units is a case in point. In general, however, expectations have been created among physicians about accuracy, certainty, and lack of ambiguity that can only be met by other technology, even if such accuracy, certainty, and lack of ambiguity are not relevant in a particular instance. Contemporary physicians tend to move to problems for which there are technological definitions or solutions.

It is not just physicians who are wooed away from the values of caring by technology. Virtually all other professional caregivers are prone to the overuse of and dependence on technology. It could hardly be otherwise since worship of technology can be found throughout Western society. The effect is to devalue caring among physicians and the public alike.

THE EFFECTS OF PRACTICE AND PAYMENT PATTERNS ON CARING

Physicians are cautioned by the Health Care Financing Administration that if they do a routine physical examination on a patient insured by Medicare they must use the code for a routine examination even if the patient has one or more serious diseases that might otherwise warrant a code with higher dollar reimbursement. If the patient has metastatic cancer, but the physician does an electrocardiogram and other tests not directly concerned with the effects of the malignancy (in a manner similar to a routine physical), the visit must be billed as a routine physical. In like manner, virtually every act that makes up medical care has been assigned a code for billing purposes. These codes are listed in *Current Procedural Terminology,* a publication put out by the American Medical Association (AMA); in 1999 the listings were revised for the fourth time (American Medical Association, 1999).

A kind of dance, or modern administrative ballet, has come into being as the Health Care Financing Administration and other third-party payers attempt to reduce costs and stop cheating by the way that they reimburse for specific codes while physicians try to maximize their incomes by creative use of the codes. It takes little imagination to see that this procedural reductionism dampens attempts to return caring to medical care. In an attempt to shift reimbursement priorities and reward primary care physicians for the activities involved in caring, the AMA added "evaluation and management" codes to *Current Procedural Terminology* in 1992: payment for technical procedures (e.g., endoscopy) was to be reduced and time spent in "cognitive" activities with patients increased. The amount of money gained by physicians was small, and the coding and documentation process was elaborate, so that less was accomplished than anticipated. In order to facilitate the shift and further reduce physicians' reliance on technical procedures, greater increases in the fees for "cognitive" services were proposed for the year 2000 (Health Care Financing Administration, 1999).

There are three straightforward ways to reduce the cost of medical care: eliminate services for which payment will be made; reduce the reimbursement for specific services; reduce the time allotted for specific services. Each of these has a direct negative impact on the ability or the motivation to care. All three methods are employed by managed care companies, Medicare, Medicaid, and other third-party payers.

In the present managed care climate, these methods have been employed to reduce the utilization and effectiveness of both the psychotherapies and physical medicine and rehabilitation. Both have traditionally been primarily involved in caring. It is of interest that one of the major contributions of the field of physical medicine and rehabilitation that developed after World War II was the importance of restoring *function,* even when structural integrity could not be restored. Effective rehabilitation involves many of the functions of caring identified by Callahan. These values have persisted in the care of persons with disabilities, but they are disvalued in the current environment. For example, for patients who have aphasia as a result of a stroke, Medicare now reimburses for speech therapy for only a short time—often insufficient time for optimal improvement. Physical therapy, when paid for at all, is often for short duration. In the past, patients with chronic musculoskeletal impairments were often maintained by long-term physical therapy; this has become impossible. As these fields contract, therapists depend less on the manual skills and relationships with patients necessary for good outcomes and more on technologies—ultrasound, muscle stimulators, and the like. As facilities and agencies try to survive despite a shrinking patient pool, the average length of a visit is changing from thirty minutes to twenty minutes. The impact on these fields is to reduce the quantity and quality of therapists. The psychotherapies and psychotherapists—psychiatrists, psychologists, and social workers, are also suffering. For both ideological and financial reasons, psychiatrists have virtually abandoned the psychotherapies in favor of psychopharmacology. Psychologists and social workers are so dominated by the requirements to shorten their treatment and justify it for managed care administrators that traditional criteria for good therapy are often abandoned. And not only is it patients and therapists who suffer: physicians, too, are deprived since they lose the model of caring that these fields promoted.

COUNTERVAILING FORCES

It is one of the contradictions of contemporary medicine that it is at once marked by the overpowering dominance of depersonalizing science and the centrality of personhood in the *person* of the patient. The beginning of the rise of the patient can probably be dated to an event in Boston in the 1920s for which Francis Peabody's famous paper "The Care of the Patient" stands as a marker (Peabody, 1927). He cites the case of a woman whose complaints of abdominal distress are investigated in the hospital without evidence of disease being discovered. She is sent home, puzzled at being told that there is nothing wrong with her although her discomfort continues unabated. In his discussion, Peabody makes it clear that it is the sick person that matters, not just the disease. He closes with the statement that "the secret of the care of the patient is in caring for the patient" (882).

The social-medicine movement of the 1930s introduced the "social history" as part of the patient's history, but the movement was pushed aside by World War II. After the war, the United States began to provide medical care across cultural boundaries in an unprecedented manner because of the devastating effects of the war on the health of populations, the resulting economic and physical ruin, and the inadequate medical resources of many nations. In the course of this, it became clear that respecting the cultural beliefs of individuals and groups was of paramount importance to the effective delivery of medical care. The rise of democracy in many parts of the world further focused on individuals and their rights. In this country, as noted above, the various rights movements and the growth of an almost radical individualism brought the person to the center of national life, including medicine. Consumerism and "patient-centered" medicine were marked by the belief that patients should be able to choose whatever they wanted from the possibilities. The corollary responsibility of physicians, in this view, was to provide all the information patients might require to make their decision. Telling the truth became the absolute standard for the provision of information, with little regard to its impact (Bok, 1978; Fox and Swazey, 1997; Jonsen, Siegler, and Winslade, 1992).

Yet, despite the increasing power of patients and the public in shaping late-twentieth-century medicine, caring continued to disappear. Why did patients not demand caring as they demanded technology, access to the latest medical advances, and specialty consultation? The most probable reason is that in a manner similar to written histories of medicine, caring has not been considered specifically a part of medicine in the sense that drug therapies or other disease-treatment modalities are. When people evaluate a physician, it may be that caring is ranked alongside other personality factors like niceness or kindness. It is not apparent to most that knowledge and skills are as vital to effective caring as they are to other aspects of medical practice. When *The Healer's Art* was published a quarter of a century ago (Cassell, 1976), its discussion of attention to the person rather than just the disease was often dismissed as referring merely to bedside manner—akin to hand holding and held in about the same regard. Medicine has progressed beyond that, but not so far that caring is seen as essential to good medicine.

It is when people become sick that they begin to appreciate that their medical care lacks (or does not lack) the caring that is so vital to their well-being. Most people, most of the time, are not sick and do not think about sickness, or they actively put the possibility of sickness from their minds. Changing the idea of medical care from *the care of the sick* to *health care* has had great public-relations and funding benefits for the health care industry, but the label serves to distract people from the idea of sickness and all that goes with it.

PALLIATIVE CARE: A MODEL

The field of palliative care medicine provides a model for how greater emphasis on caring might be restored in medical care. Palliative care has its origins in the modern hospice movement founded by Dame Cicely Saunders in England (see Saunders and Kastenbaum, 1997). Built on the tradition of the religious institution of hospice as a place of shelter and care for the dying, the modern hospice brought together a number of elements: a medical understanding of pain and symptom control; new insights into grief and loss; recognition of the spiritual and transcendent dimensions of care; and incorporation of the family into the unit of care. Hospice theory starts with acknowledgment that curative medicine has failed the dying patient. Hospice caregivers, in contradistinction to many hospital physicians, understand the importance of the relief of the symptoms that come to form the dying person's active illness. Thus, the relief of pain became an early goal of hospice medicine. Experience with the dying reveals that their distress is not solely due to physical symptoms, so Saunders emphasized that the care of the dying requires attention to emotional and spiritual needs as well as the physical. Their suffering, like all suffering, can involve any aspect of the person. In fact, suffering is a special distress, separate from its physical, emotional, or spiritual sources within the patient. Because of its origins within each patient, it is always personal, individual, and lonely. Accordingly, its relief—which can be accomplished even when lifting the burden of the physical illness is impossible—must be directed at the person by the person of the caregiver. Impersonal, technical, or mechanical care fails to address suffering. It is a common experience that when suffering itself is addressed, the amount and kinds of medications required to relieve pain are much less than when pain alone is treated.

A significant element in the history of the modern hospice was its removal from mainstream medicine. When Saint Christopher's Hospice opened in England in 1967, it was a completely new building, freestanding and funded outside the National Health Service. Significantly, patients moved out of the hospital system to the hospice as inpatients or outpatients (a situation that holds in the United States today). The hospice was seen as a haven from the neglect, abandonment, and lack of care that dying patients were experiencing as people who were no longer curable, stranded in a system focused on the cure of disease.

In the United States, for decades the hospice movement was on the margins of medicine. The hospice message of total care, concern with suffering, aggressive symptom relief, and attention to families as well as patients seemed to have little or no impact on medical education, hospital practice, or day-to-day medical care. Within the hospice movement itself, the importance of caring was central: hospices were usually run by nurses dedicated to the total care of their patients. Active volunteer programs and philanthropic funds supported the mission. And, around the world and over the years, those caregivers—nurses, social workers, physicians, and others dedicated to the care of the dying—formed a close-knit community.

With specialization, increasing numbers of physicians have become specifically knowledgeable about pain relief and other treatment modalities. Palliative care as a specialty has blossomed and new journals have appeared. At one time in recent years, as public attention to proper symptom relief and care of the dying grew and widespread acceptance of methods for adequate pain relief was evidenced, it appeared that the hospice movement's central message of caring would have a major impact on medicine. Unfortunately, this does not appear to have happened, at least up to the present. In the United Kingdom, Canada, Australia, and New Zealand, it is true, specialized training programs have become common and palliative care departments have been formed in many hospitals. In the United States, despite the fact that Medicare funds hospice care (see Moore and McCollough, 2000) and that pain-treatment programs have become common, true palliative care as a part of hospitals is unusual. Rather, the field of palliative care seems to be in danger (and not only in the United States) of retreating from its acceptance of the importance of treating every aspect of the patient—"body, mind, and spirit."

The focus now is increasingly on pain and symptom management. On retiring after five years as editor of *Progress in Palliative Care,* a major journal in the field, Dr. Sam Ahmedzai reviewed recent developments in the field. He comments on an author writing about the spiritual aspects of helping patients confront death and then writes, critically, "The view now, within palliative medicine, is that it is okay to be a symptomatologist—and proud of it!" (1997: 236). Ahmedzai concludes that while the relief of suffering directly related to symptoms is important, other sources of suffering are not the business of palliative care.

WHAT CAN BE DONE?

The forces that keep caring from being a central concern of medical practice—the advance of science and technology, the values conveyed in graduate and postgraduate medical education, and patient demands—are formidable and pervasive. Seeing palliative care medicine retreat from caring, the foundation of its origins, and the necessity for its patients, should be sobering.

A return to caring will not be accomplished without acknowledging and aggressively addressing the factors that continue to drive it out of medicine. My belief is that until the person (whether sick or well), rather than the disease, is the object and subject of medicine, the goal will not be achieved. Caring is not addressed only at the psychological, social, or spiritual needs of patients; it is aimed at the person in whom these dimensions are found. Caring, like the relief of suffering, must be personal. This cannot take place—save by exceptionally gifted individuals—in the absence of trained and disciplined knowledge of *person* as there is now knowledge of *body*.

A medicine of caring, to have important impact, cannot depend on those who are especially compassionate. It must be part of the practice of ordinary physicians and other caregivers. It may be possible to form special educational programs in medical schools or hospitals that will graduate caring physicians. But these individuals will regress to the mean—failing the ideals taught to them, through no fault of their own—unless the foundational impediments to caring discussed in the beginning of this chapter are confronted.

The exclusivity of biological science in medical education and medicine requires redress. Medical (biological) science is absolutely vital to human progress, but it is only one of the kinds of knowledge that doctors require. Medical educators are horrified by the thought that hard biological science must be pushed from the center of the medical-school curriculum to make way for the other human sciences—for other ways of understanding the human condition. It is a demand that some educators have been making—to no avail—for a generation. If this demand horrifies the medical education establishment, it is probably correct. The analogy may seem harsh, but the current hegemony of hard science is reminiscent of the long reign of the Scholastics. From before the eleventh century and well into the fourteenth century, the schoolmen, the Scholastics, with their origins in the universities of Paris and Oxford, ruled philosophy and theology and imposed their views on the world. Everything in nature, in their worldview—indeed, everything in the world—served only to illustrate the place of God and the importance of theology in the universe, a theology in which views of orthodoxy were rigidly controlled. The Scholastics brought reason into the thinking of a previously semibarbarous world. It was, however, a reason subject to unblinking authority. When Roger Bacon published his belief in the importance of experimental science for understanding nature (ideas that seem mild to us today) he paid for it with years of house arrest (Taylor, 1966).

The problem of changing the nature of medical education is daunting. Change that is less than well thought out, necessarily almost radical change, will surely fail and join the parade of the disappointing starts of the past—for example, the brief career of the attempts to teach behavioral science in medical education. It does not have to happen at many schools. One school will do, just as was the case when Johns Hopkins led the United States into the world of scientific medical education.

Another alternative is to emulate the early days of the hospice movement, when a principled kind of medicine based in the real needs of the sick generated a small group of training programs around the country (and the world). The very fact of the uniqueness of programs for restoring the importance of caring will serve to separate them from mainstream medicine and thus generate a cohesive community among their adherents. The training will be different than current graduate and postgraduate education because it will actively teach the skills necessary to take care of sick (and well) persons. Much of this knowledge and many of these skills have previously been subsumed under the rubric of the art of medicine. It is often presumed that this art can only be learned by experiencing patients under the guidance of proper role models. How such nonsense continues to be spread is a mystery. The word *art* in this sense comes from the Greek *techne,* which is art like that of crafts (tinsmithing), not the fine arts. One could further argue that even the fine arts are taught sufficiently for novices to develop their skills. Yet, papers continue to be published that make the same mistake, implying that the art of caring cannot be actively taught.

Finally, there are no longer enough role models. Time, money, and committed people will be required to develop the curricular materials necessary to teach caring. We should never forget that medical students still enter medical school because they want to take care of people. Their training, the intellectual environment, and too many societal pressures steal away the ability, but not the underlying desire. The need to care flows from sick patients, wherever they are. We must reignite the desire *and provide the training* so that physicians can return to their fundamental calling. "Into whatsoever houses I enter, I will enter to help the sick."

REFERENCES

Ahmedzai, S. (1997). Five years, five threads. *Progress in Palliative Care* 5: 235–37.

Albutt, T. C. (1911). Medicine. In *Encyclopedia Britannica,* vol. 18.

American Medical Association (1999). *Current Procedural Terminology.* 4th ed. Chicago: American Medical Association.

Bardes, C. L. (1998). Evaluating the curriculum with standardized patients. *Academic Medicine* 73: 626–27.

Beauchamp, T. L., and Childress, J. F. (1994). *Principles of Biomedical Ethics.* 4th ed. New York: Oxford University Press.

Bok, S. (1978). *Lying: Moral Choice in Public and Private Life.* New York: Pantheon.

Cassell, E. J. (1976). *The Healer's Art.* New York: Lippincott.

Cassell, E. J. (1993). The sorcerer's broom: Medicine's rampant technology. *Hastings Center Report* 23: 32–39.

Childress, J. F. (1982). *Who Should Decide? Paternalism in Health Care.* New York: Oxford University Press.

Coulter, H. L. (1988). *Divided Legacy: Origins of Modern Western Medicine—J. B. Van Helmont to Claude Bernard.* Washington, DC: Wehawken Books.

Fox, R. C., and Swazey, J. P. (1997). Medical morality is not bioethics. In N. S. Jecker, A. R. Jonsen, and R. A. Pearlman, eds., *Bioethics: An Introduction to the History, Methods, and Practice.* Boston: Jones & Bartlett.

Health Care Financing Administration (New York Region) (1999). *2000 Medicare Participation Enrollment Package.* Crompond, NY: Empire Medicare Services.

Jonsen, A. R., Siegler, M., and Winslade, W. J. (1992). *Clinical Ethics.* 3rd ed. New York: McGraw-Hill.

King, L. S. (1978). *The Philosophy of Medicine: The Early Eighteenth Century.* Cambridge: Harvard University Press.

Kramer, A. M. (1996). Demography and health status. In D. W. Jahnigen and R. W. Schrier, eds., *Geriatric Medicine,* 2nd. ed., pp. 18–27. Cambridge: Blackwell Science.

Moore, P. C., and McCollough, R. H. (2000). Hospice: End-of-life care at home. In R. H. Binstock and L. E. Cluff, eds., *Home Care Advances: Essential Research and Policy Issues,* pp. 101–16. New York: Springer Publishing.

Peabody, F. W. (1927). The care of the patient. *Journal of the American Medical Association* 88: 877–82.

Pirsig, R. M. (1979). *Zen and the Art of Motorcycle Maintenance: An Inquiry into Values.* New York: Morrow Quill Paperback.

Rothman, D. J. (1991). *Strangers at the Bedside.* New York: Basic Books.

Saunders, C., and Kastenbaum, R. (1997). *Hospice Care on the International Scene.* New York: Springer Publishing.

Schneider, C. E. (1998). *The Practice of Autonomy: Patients, Doctors, and Medical Decisions.* New York: Oxford University Press.

Taylor, H. O. (1966). *The Medieval Mind: A History of the Development of Thought and Emotion in the Middle Ages.* 4th ed., vol. 2. Cambridge: Harvard University Press.

Wilkins, R., ed. (1991). *The Doctor's Quotations Book.* New York: Barnes & Noble.

6

Caring and Medical Education

KENNETH M. LUDMERER, M.D.,
AND RENÉE C. FOX, PH.D.

A LONGSTANDING assumption in medical education is that caring, like factual medical knowledge, can be taught through the medical curriculum. Since World War II, this assumption has given rise to a series of efforts to introduce various nontechnical subjects into the curriculum; for example, the behavioral sciences and medical history in the 1950s and 1960s, and the medical humanities (including literature, art, and music) and bioethics in the 1970s, 1980s, and 1990s (Ludmerer, 1999). Most recently, many schools have demonstrated a renewed interest in "white coat" ceremonies for matriculating medical students as a means of fostering professionalism and caring (Swick et al., 1999).

There is little doubt that formal instruction can help physicians become effectively caring and compassionate. A number of important concepts from the social sciences are central to understanding the whole patient. Examples include the distinction between disease and illness, the notion of the social construction of clinical reality, and the concept of suffering and its relation to organic illness (Cassell, 1982; Kleinman, Eisenberg, and Good, 1978). Communication skills can be improved with coaching and feedback, particularly in encounters with patients from cultural and socioeconomic backgrounds different from those of the interviewing physician (Novack, Drossman, and Lipkin, 1993). Tools of the behavioral sciences can be used to improve patients' adherence to medical prescriptions—for instance, by teaching students to prescribe a drug once a day when possible, rather than several times a day. Most important, empathy involves the ability to understand things from another person's point of view. This provides a cogent argument for introducing courses in the social sciences and humanities, whose fundamental intellectual skills involve the projection of the self into another perspective.

Nevertheless, a common error of medical educators has been to regard formal course work as "intellectual magic bullets" for cultivating caring attitudes without considering the broad social and cultural milieu in which caring and compassion are shaped (Fox, 1990: 204). Numerous sociological studies over the past five decades have documented the profound impact of the entire institutional environment of the academic health center on the attitudes, values, beliefs, modes of thought, and behavior of medical students (Fox, 1989). In the broad view of the professionalization process (often called the socialization process) that has emerged from this work, attitudes are seen to be shaped by the totality of students' interactions in laboratories, classrooms, wards, and clinics with faculty, house officers, patients, hospital staff, and one another. Accordingly, formal course work must be considered only one of the many factors that affect the development of caring. Indeed, a harsh, unfriendly institutional culture can undermine course work on caring. For instance, the effects of a brilliant lecture on caring to the assembled medical class can easily be undone should students return to a ward culture where, for example, residents routinely speak of the GOMERS (GOMER—"Get Out of My Emergency Room!"—a derogatory term in the argot of house officers for an elderly or critically ill patient who has just been admitted).

In this context, because of changes in the culture of academic health centers that implicitly undermine the values that medical educators wish to teach, we are concerned about the ability of today's students and house officers to become caring physicians. An "erosion of caring" has occurred in the U.S. health care system, and this phenomenon has penetrated the walls of academic health centers. The fact that many academic health centers are not only caught up in a spiral of market-oriented competition but are struggling for financial survival intensifies this situation (Ludmerer, 1999). As a result, the milieu in which medical students are undergoing their professional education and socialization has been adversely affected. The new teaching environment fundamentally contradicts the ideal principles of solicitous medical care, thus making it much more difficult to transmit these principles to physicians in training. No matter what the content and emphasis of the formal curriculum may be, students and house staff are continually exposed to latent "messages" about caring that emanate from the "reality" of how care is delivered in the academic health center—messages that often run counter to what medical educators are trying and hoping to convey about caring.

In this chapter, we review the challenges to caring in today's health care environment and describe how the internal culture of academic health centers no longer readily reinforces the values and principles of caring that medical educators wish to impart. In this discussion, we make two overarching points. The first is that a significant part of the teaching and learning of caring takes place implicitly, in ways that are not didactically a part of the curriculum and that are not always intended or recognized by educators. The second is that the teaching of caring cannot be properly considered outside of the organizational, institutional, social, and cultural conditions within which such teaching takes place. Ultimately, educators will have their best chance at producing caring doctors only if they succeed in restoring the internal culture of academic health centers so that it is once again less commercial and more caring.

THE EROSION OF CARING IN MEDICAL PRACTICE

Our conception of caring is premised on the notion of "competent caring" and "caring competence" (Fox, 1990). In this definition of caring, scientific and technical competence are integral parts. We agree with Walsh McDermott, the eminent internist, medical scientist, and humanist, who wrote, "If I were terribly ill it would be all right to get me a physician who knew all about the 'whole man,' but I wished to be damn sure he 'knew about my parts'" (McDermott, 1979).

However, technical competence alone does not result in caring. Qualities such as empathy, compassion, kindness, and open and dignified communication with patients and their families are also indispensable. This aspect of caring was well described by Philip A. Tumulty, a distinguished clinician and medical teacher from Johns Hopkins, who pointed out that management of a sick person only begins with making a diagnosis and prescribing a treatment. "Management," he wrote, "means that the physician comprehends and is sensitive to the total effects of an illness on the total person, the spiritual effects as well as the physical, and the social as well as the economic" (Tumulty, 1978: 21).

The fundamental prerequisite for caring is for physicians (and other health care workers) to have sufficient time with their patients. Good medical care simply cannot be provided on the fly. Problem solving—

figuring out a diagnosis, or determining the best treatment for the individual patient—requires time for physicians to think and reflect. Similarly, thoroughness and attention to detail require enough time for physicians to listen attentively and examine patients carefully. Doctors also need time to get to know patients, determine individual wishes and preferences, provide education and counseling, teach about ways to prevent illness and promote health, address psychosocial concerns, and provide comfort and compassion. It should also be noted that patients, particularly when troubled by sensitive issues, may not immediately blurt out their questions or concerns. Time is often required for patients to become sufficiently at ease to bring up what is really bothering them. Tumulty (1978) observed that physicians' "greatest assets" are their "ability to listen and to talk" (20). This, of course, requires time.

In this context, the great threat to caring in today's health care environment, driven as it is by economics, is that time, in the name of efficiency, is being squeezed out of patient care. Managed care organizations, with their insistence on maximizing the "throughput" of patients (seeing as many patients as possible, as quickly as possible), have been forcing doctors to churn through patients in assembly-line fashion at ever-accelerating rates of speed. In 1990, fifteen to twenty office patients a day was considered pushing the limit for an internist or family physician who wanted to provide quality care; today, forty to fifty are common, and reports of seventy or more are not unheard of (Lowes, 1995). In 1997, doctors on average spent eight minutes talking to each patient, less than half as much time as a decade before (Goldberg, 1997). That might be enough time to treat healthy patients who have no more than a cold or sprained ankle, but it is hardly enough time to allow doctors to evaluate, treat, counsel, and comfort patients with the broad range of illnesses that appear in American society today.

Evidence has also been accumulating that patients are often dissatisfied with their care when office visits are perceived as too short. A variety of studies have reiterated what clinicians, humanists, and social scientists have long known: that patient satisfaction depends heavily on good communication, a caring, attentive doctor, and a thorough explanation of the patient's condition and treatment. When physician time is in short supply, these goals are seldom achieved and patients are often unhappy with their care (Froehlich and Welch, 1996; Howie et al., 1991; Laine et al., 1996; Ridsdale et al., 1989; Rubin et al., 1993; Waitzkin, 1984). A stereotype has begun to emerge of the doctor, hand already on the examining room doorknob when greeting a patient, using body language to encourage the patient to leave even before the consultation has begun. Advice columnist Ann Landers observed that the most frequent complaint she receives from her readers about doctors is "the feeling that they are not getting enough of their doctor's time" (Landers, 1993). It has also been suggested that the growing popularity of alternative medicine in the 1990s could be explained in part by the fact that its practitioners have more time to give to patients (Davidoff, 1997).

The quality of caring in hospital settings is also dependent on the human interactions between patients and hospital workers—not only doctors, nurses, and other health care professionals, but also nonmedical personnel like housekeepers, blood drawers, and transporters. There is much that employees even seemingly uninvolved with patient care can do to make hospitalization a caring experience for patients. For instance, housekeepers can greet patients with a warm smile and friendly conversation and provide assistance with the telephone or getting comfortable in bed. Historically, it has been the totality of the institutional environment that has determined the level of "caring" a hospital has been able to provide for its patients (Rosenberg, 1987).

At the turn of the century, as hospitals have come under increasingly severe financial pressures, the level of caring they have been able to provide has also diminished. This has resulted from the downsizing—severe cuts in personnel—that they have been forced to undertake in order to combat the markedly lower payments they now receive from third-party payers. Many hospitals are operating with staffs less than half the size of a decade ago. Nurses and other professional staff members have experienced the most dramatic reductions in numbers, but most groups of hospital workers have been similarly affected. Housekeepers, with twice the number of rooms to clean, have little time to be kind to patients, lest their pay be docked for being "unproductive" (not cleaning as many rooms as possible, as quickly as possible). Many hospitals aggressively compete for patients by advertising the television sets and carpeting they have put in, but that does not alter the fact that they have become less caring places because there are too few personnel to attend to the medical and personal needs of patients.

Kenneth Ludmerer, one of the authors of this chapter, recently witnessed the effects of hospital downsizing while caring for a patient at a respected teaching hospital. An eighty-five-year-old woman had soiled herself in bed because no one had responded to her request for help with the bedpan. The nurses and orderlies were neither lazy nor unconcerned. Rather, the floor was full, the patients were sick, and staffing was at half the level it had been a few years before. Events like this do not show up in a hospital's mortality statistics, but they do illustrate how financial pressures on hospitals have contributed to their becoming less caring institutions.

THE EROSION OF CARING IN MEDICAL EDUCATION

Throughout the twentieth century, medical schools in the United States have found themselves with two homes—one in the university, the other in the health care delivery system. Of the two, the ties to the university have traditionally been far stronger. Since the passage of the Medicare and Medicaid legislation in 1965, however, the patient-care activities of medical faculties have grown enormously, and the ties of medical schools to the health care delivery system have correspondingly increased. As a result, academic health centers today operate in the "real world" of health care delivery. Driven by intense, market-oriented competition, they are under great pressure to see as many patients as possible, both inpatients and outpatients (Ludmerer, 1999). This state of affairs has had subversive effects on the ability of medical faculties to impart caring attitudes and behaviors to learners; it affects even their being able to teach the fundamentals of clinical care.

One consequence of current market forces on medical schools has been the fact that fewer and fewer clinical faculty are available to serve as teachers and mentors. Instead, today's faculty are under intense pressure to be "clinically productive"—that is, to see as many paying patients as possible so that they can help keep the academic medical center financially afloat. (It is of note that the common definition of *clinical productivity* at medical schools refers to the amount of professional fees generated, not the quantity or quality of care. Ordinary care delivered to paying patients is considered being clinically productive; outstanding care given to charity patients is not.) Ludmerer has heard the chairman of internal medicine at a prestigious medical school tell his faculty in all seriousness, "If you want to teach, do so at lunch—and keep your lunches short." Because of such pressures, clinical faculty members today have little time to teach, advise, or serve as mentors. In addition, medical students and house staff have dwindling opportunities to observe faculty doctoring in a teacherly, caring way (Ludmerer, 1999).

A second consequence of the competitive era has been changes in the ambience of teaching institutions. These changes have had problematic effects on the teaching and learning of caring. At present, hospitalized patients consist primarily of two types: one group is admitted for very short stays (frequently for less than one day); the other consists of gravely ill patients in intensive care units. In neither case are students and house staff able to get to know their patients well or observe and learn techniques of empathy and good patient communication. In the ambulatory clinics of teaching hospitals, patients are being seen in droves in a pass-through way so that "throughput" can be maximized. Since education gets in the way of "throughput," students in outpatient offices are typically reduced to being passive observers. Students often observe attending physicians cut corners in the management of patients and communicate with their patients in a hurried fashion, if at all (Ludmerer, 1999).

Because of such conditions, many medical faculties have become demoralized. They have been troubled at being unable to teach medicine and take care of patients in a way that fulfills their criteria of clinical and moral excellence. In particular, they have bemoaned the new rules of faculty practice that insist on maximum "clinical productivity" because those rules have interfered with teaching and patient care and with the instillation of a caring spirit in learners. "We don't see how we can be educators," one pediatrics professor said of current conditions (quoted in Mangan, 1996: A18).

Many medical schools have responded to present conditions with renewed attempts to instill caring and professionalism among medical students. However, most of these efforts have concentrated on traditional curricular methods (Swick et al., 1999). Few schools have come squarely to grips with the contradiction between the principles of caring they wish to impart and the reality of the existing organization and conditions of care in which their students learn medicine. Medical educators have seldom pondered the potential long-term consequences of educating the nation's physicians in today's commercial atmosphere—one in which the good visit is a short visit, patients are "consumers," and institutional officials speak more often of the financial balance sheet than of service and the relief of suffering. It is imperative that medical educators begin to consider these issues since the present environment does little to validate the altruism and idealism that students typically bring with them to the study of medicine.

SOME SOCIOLOGICAL QUESTIONS

Though it is clear that the teaching and learning of caring is presently occurring in a highly commercial environment that undermines the principles instructors wish to instill, a number of important sociological questions remain unanswered. These require further exploration—not just speculatively, but through the gathering of relevant data.

First, we need detailed studies to describe precisely what today's medical students and house officers are latently learning about care and caring from the hospital milieu to which they are exposed. What exactly are they seeing, hearing, and experiencing through their interaction with the current impersonalized setting of health care delivery and their interaction (or lack of interaction) with faculty? Similarly, studies of medical teachers are also needed to examine how they are being affected, attitudinally and behaviorally, by the current contexts of medical care and education. What messages are teachers communicating to learners, both intentionally and inadvertently?

Second, we need to know much more about the personality and motivation of today's medical students. For instance, what has led them to become physicians in this era of ferment in American medicine? What attitudes and values are they bringing into the process of becoming a physician? What conceptions do they have of being a physician—of what medical practice should be like and what it will be like? What do they know and think about "managed care"? What effect has the considerable amount of volunteer, community activity in which they have characteristically engaged had on them? What sort of experiences have they had vis-à-vis illness?

Much information of a quantitative sort has been gathered about medical students. We know where today's students were born, where they were raised, and where they attended college. We also know their college majors, college grades, scores on the Medical College Admissions Test, parental occupations and income, and racial, religious, and gender distribution. Thus, we have learned that medical students are still largely from the upper-middle class, Caucasian, and frequently sons or daughters of physicians (a high level of occupational inheritance). Men and women now enter medical school in nearly equal numbers.

However, it is extraordinary how little medical educators know in a qualitative way about medical students. Demographic facts do not tell us "who" the students are attitudinally, what their sense of being a physician is, or how they are like or unlike their predecessors in medicine. We know little about their reasons for choosing medicine as a career, what they hope to derive from it, and what they aspire to contribute in return. Medical educators have typically been too prone to suppose that, in these respects, they "know" the young women and men whom they are teaching.

Last, we know little about the consequences of the present ferment in American medicine on who will select medical careers in the future. It is hard not to be enthusiastic about today's students, who are not only bright and motivated but who have chosen to enter medicine despite knowing that physician incomes in the future are likely to be lower than in the past. This suggests that they have chosen medicine for the right reasons—intellectual excitement and the opportunities to help fellow human beings. However, what if present trends continue unabated, and external pressures force medicine to become a less caring profession? In such a scenario, it is not at all clear what talents and capacity for caring students will bring with them into the study of medicine or what will happen to these propensities and abilities en route to their becoming physicians.

THE CHALLENGES AHEAD

Perhaps the most important sociological lesson for medical education is that teaching and learning are not necessarily symmetrical. A great deal of what students and house officers learn does not come from the formal curriculum. Rather, it occurs in an unplanned, informal, latent way, catalyzed and conveyed by the time period, institutional setting, and social and cultural climate in which their professional education and socialization take place.

In this context, the greatest need for the teaching of caring to medical students and house officers is modification of the internal culture of the academic health center so that it better reinforces the values that medical educators wish to impart. At present, this represents no small task, for the managed care revolution has caused medical schools and teaching hospitals to become much less friendly to patients and students than they were even a few years ago. Nevertheless, until the internal culture of academic health centers can be made less commercial and more service-oriented, our efforts to produce caring physicians will continue to be undermined.

Ultimately, the fate of medical education in general and of efforts to teach caring in particular will depend upon what happens to the health care delivery system. There is nothing new in this, for medical schools in the United States have always depended on having a health care delivery system willing to supply them with patients, financial resources, and moral and political support (Ludmerer, 1985, 1999). If the country is able to create a health care delivery system in the twenty-first century that allows doctors enough time to heal, teachers enough time to teach, and learners enough time to learn, then medical education will find itself in good shape. Conversely, if the country fails to achieve a delivery system with those qualities, then the quality of medical education, particularly that of the teaching of caring, will continue to suffer. Indeed, it can be argued that if the conditions of medical practice remain harsh, it will not matter even if medical schools succeed in teaching caring and good patient communication. As Roger Bulger, president of the Association of Academic Health Centers has written, "Students who may have been taught all of the best techniques for communicating with patients will soon learn to ignore those techniques if their practice environment discourages such behavior by, for example, requiring them to see a different patient every ten minutes" (Bulger, 1992: 262).

There is reason to hope that, ultimately, a system of health care delivery will be created that will allow doctors to continue to learn about and practice caring medicine. Such a system will not evolve automatically, but it can be accomplished if medical leaders have the courage to address the structural problems confronting medical education and practice directly and are willing to stand up for the interests of patients and the public. The general principles to follow have already been identified (Ludmerer, 1999; Sullivan, 1999). Society, patients, and the medical profession will be well served by such an effort.

ACKNOWLEDGMENT

Dr. Ludmerer's work was supported in part by a grant from the Charles E. Culpeper Foundation.

REFERENCES

Bulger, R. J. (1992). Responding to incentives in academic health centers. *Health Affairs* 11(4): 261–62.

Cassell, E. J. (1982). The nature of suffering and the goals of medicine. *New England Journal of Medicine* 306: 639–45.

Davidoff, F. (1997). Time. *Annals of Internal Medicine* 127: 485.

Epstein, A. M., Taylor, W. C., and Seage, G. R., III (1985). Effects of patients' socioeconomic status and physicians' training and practice on patient-doctor communication. *American Journal of Medicine* 78: 101–6.

Fox, R. C. (1989). *The Sociology of Medicine: A Participant-Observer's View.* Englewood Cliffs, NJ: Prentice-Hall.

Fox, R. C. (1990). Training in caring competence: The perennial problem in North American medical education. In H. C. Hendrie and C. Lloyd, eds., *Educating Competent and Humane Physicians*, pp. 199–216. Bloomington: Indiana University Press.

Froehlich, G. W., and Welch, H. G. (1996). Meeting walk-in patients' expectations for testing. *Journal of General Internal Medicine* 11: 470–74.

Goldberg, R. (1997). What's happened to the healing process? *Wall Street Journal*, June 18: A22.

Howie, J. G., Porter, A. M. D., Heaney, D. G., and Hopton, J. L. (1991). Long to short consultation ratio: A proxy measure of quality of care for general practice. *British Journal of General Practice* 41: 48–54.

Kleinman, A., Eisenberg, L., and Good, B. (1978). Culture, illness, and care: Clinical lessons from anthropological and cross-cultural research. *Annals of Internal Medicine* 88: 251–58.

Laine, C., Davidoff, F., Lewis, C. F., Nelson, E. C., Nelson E., Kessler, R. C., and Delbanco, T. (1996). Important elements of outpatient care: A comparison of patients' and physicians' opinions. *Annals of Internal Medicine* 125: 640–45.

Landers, W. (1993). What patients want. *Harvard Medical Alumni Bulletin* 67 (autumn): 42–43.

Lowes, R. L. (1995). Are you expected to see too many patients? *Medical Economics* 27 (March): 52–59.

Ludmerer, K. M. (1985). *Learning to Heal: The Development of American Medical Education.* New York: Basic Books.

Ludmerer, K. M. (1999). *Time to Heal: American Medical Education from the Turn of the Century to the Era of Managed Care.* New York: Oxford University Press.

Mangan, K. S. (1996). Medical schools are reining in the salaries of faculty members. *Chronicle of Higher Education,* July 26: A18.

McDermott, W. (1979). Letter to Alexander G. Bearn. January 24, folder 8, box 22, Walsh McDermott Papers, Archives. New York: New York Hospital–Cornell Medical Center.

Novack, D. H., Drossman, D. A., and Lipkin, M., Jr. (1993). Medical interviewing and interpersonal skills teaching in U.S. medical schools. *Journal of the American Medical Association* 269: 2101–5.

Ridsdale, L., Carruthers, M., Morris, R., and Ridsdale, J. (1989). Study of the effect of time availability on the consultation. *Journal of the Royal College of General Practitioners* 39: 488–91.

Rosenberg, C. E. (1987). *The Care of Strangers: The Rise of America's Hospital System.* New York: Basic Books.

Rubin, H. R., Gandek, B., Rogers, W. H., Kosinski, M., McHorney C. A., and Ware, J. E., Jr. (1993). Patients' ratings of outpatient visits in different practice settings: Results from the medical outcomes study. *Journal of the American Medical Association* 270: 835–40.

Sullivan, W. M. (1999). What is left of professionalism after managed care? *Hastings Center Report* 29(2): 7–13.

Swick, H. M., Szenas, P., Danoff, D., and Whitcomb, M. E. (1999). Teaching professionalism in undergraduate medical education. *Journal of the American Medical Association* 282: 830–32.

Tumulty, P. A. (1978). What is a clinician and what does he do? *New England Journal of Medicine* 283: 20–24.

Waitzkin, H. (1984). Doctor-patient communication. *Journal of the American Medical Association* 252: 2441–46.

7

Caring in Institutional Settings

MATHY MEZEY, ED.D., R.N., F.A.A.N.,
AND CLAIRE FAGIN, PH.D., R.N., F.A.A.N.

> Some anthropologists have concluded that the first real sign of civilization, rather than man-made tools, is of healed bone fractures, because they indicate that the human being was fed and attended to until recovery could occur.
>
> P. Benner, in *Nursing and Health Care Perspectives,* 1999

WHETHER IN hospitals or nursing homes, how health care is delivered matters. Despite growth in home care, people with severe acute illness, recurrent and progressive chronic illness, and severe functional and mental frailty continue to require care in acute care and long-term care institutions.

Patients entering these health care institutions expect to be "cared for" in a humane manner. Yet, more than ever, patients and family members worry about the extent to which hospitals and nursing homes "care" about them as individuals, represent "caring" environments, and offer "quality of care." Despite major advances in technology, patients often view services rendered in health care settings as uncaring and, thus, inadequate. In fact, patients and families typically find themselves in adversarial positions when dealing with caregivers and administrative staff in hospitals and nursing homes: pleading with nurses for pain medication; ambushing physicians for information; and tangling with financial services departments over medical bills.

In their advertisements and commercials, hospitals and nursing homes tout modern imaging technology or a new physical plant as evidence of quality care. For patients and family members, however, what reflects "kind and humane" health care are caring and a caring environment—attention in which providers and the institution convey a sense of (to quote the 1995 *Oxford English Dictionary's* definition of *caring*) "concern and interest." From the patients' points of view, the knowledge *and* the warmth of personnel in the hospital admissions office, the clinical grasp of nurses to identify impending problems, the nurses' speed in responding to a call bell, and the competence of physicians *and* their willingness to sit down while explaining a test result—all these *together* represent caring, a caring environment, and quality of care.

To a great extent, when people talk about "care" in health care institutions, they are talking about nursing care. Nursing practice has been central in the development and evolution of hospitals and nursing homes (Risse, 1999). With the emergence of the modern hospital and nursing home, nurses have been the principle providers charged with the responsibility of creating a "caring" environment that considers both a patient's illness and the patient's responses to that illness. Nurses and nursing personnel are by far the largest group of providers employed by hospitals and nursing homes. Unfortunately, in today's hospitals and nursing homes, nurses increasingly share patients' concerns about lapses in care and the failure to create a caring environment.

This chapter describes the emergence of the modern hospital and nursing home and the important role of nurses in caring for patients in these settings and delineates contemporary forces that make it difficult for nurses to fulfill their caring responsibilities. The chapter closes with a discussion of the challenges involved in protecting and enhancing the substructure and superstructure of caring in the fragile environments that currently characterize our health care institutions.

HOSPITALS

Institutions for the care of the sick and disabled changed dramatically toward the end of the nineteenth century and further changed during the last half of the twentieth century. Nineteenth-century hospitals served mostly to house poor persons who were sick, destitute, and dying. They were charitable institutions, established by religious orders, through philanthropy, or with public funds. Toward the end of the nineteenth century, however, when anesthetics and antiseptic procedures were introduced, patients went to hospitals to get well, rather than to die. The presence of trained nurses helped people appreciate that hospitals were caring institutions worthy of their trust and their care (Shryock, 1936).

Concern about the care provided in many hospitals early in the twentieth century led the American College of Surgeons, in 1913, to develop strict requirements for hospitals and their physicians. In 1918, only 13 percent of hospitals were approved by the college. By 1932, however, 93 percent of large hospitals were approved, leading to regular inspection and evaluation of the structure and procedures of hospitals to ensure the adequacy of their facilities, technology, services, and professional staff (Shryock, 1936).

Until well after World War II, hospital services for the poor and medically indigent were provided in large wards often housing twelve to forty patients crowded together with little or no privacy. Facilities for bathing and toileting were limited, if available at all. Hospitals still relied on charitable contributions and local governments to cover the cost of care. Patients who were able to pay for their care had some measure of privacy in rooms accommodating from one to four patients. Attention to the amenities of care was an expression of caring for personal needs. Nurses were readily available and private nursing could be obtained, thus providing attention to patients' requests for comfort, support, information, counseling, and personal services.

The modern hospital emerged in response to advances in medical technology that greatly improved the diagnosis and treatment of disease. With almost unlimited financing from federal construction funds, Medicare, Medicaid, and private health care insurance, hospitals responded by developing better and larger facilities, increasing professional and administrative staff, adding more sophisticated technology, and meeting the interest and demand of increasing numbers of middle-class patients for more attractive, homelike or hotel-like facilities. In part, these changes were attributable to competition between hospitals wanting to attract referring physicians and patients. Improvements in amenities also allowed hospitals to appeal to the caring and personal needs and interests of their patients. Private rooms made it possible for a member of the patient's family to remain in the room during the day or night, providing companionship and helping to ensure that appropriate care by hospital personnel was provided.

Facilities, however, in and of themselves do not substitute for personal attention from hospital personnel, particularly from nurses and physicians. In more recent times, attempts to control escalating costs have markedly changed hospital staffing and patient services. When hospitals were fully reimbursed to cover costs, staffing of hospital services was generous. In fact, there were occasions when it was difficult for hospitals to fill all nursing vacancies. But when hospital costs escalated to a degree unacceptable to Medicare, Medicaid, and private insurers, cost-control measures that began to be implemented in the 1980s markedly reduced days of hospitalization and patients were discharged earlier to their homes, to nursing homes, or to rehabilitation facilities. Because they were unable to keep patient beds occupied, hospitals downsized, closing beds and reducing personnel, especially middle-management nurses. The number of hospital beds in the nation decreased from 6 beds per 1,000 population in 1980 to 3.24 per 1,000 in 1997. Interestingly, however, the number of personnel employed in the nation's hospitals increased from 329 per 100 patients in 1980 to 467 per 100 in 1997 (American Hospital Association, 1999). Much of this increase can be attributed to the enormous growth in medical technology, which required additional technical personnel, other personnel needed to manage the business side of hospitals, and additional services such as intensive care units.

These contemporary changes in hospital operations, staffing, and facilities are particularly worrisome because patients in hospitals are sicker overall than was the case in the past. With the population aging, and the number of persons aged seventy-five and over growing rapidly, hospitalized patients are, on average, getting older. In 1996, for example, the number of days of care of discharged hospitalized patients over seventy-five years of age was about twice that of those aged sixty-five to seventy-four, and five times that of the population aged forty-five to sixty-four (*Statistical Abstract of the United States,* 1998). Patients with chronic diseases and their associated complications and acute exacerbations fill most medical and surgical beds. Caring for these patients requires special skills and a special kind of knowledge and understanding. This need emphasizes the importance of training in care of the aged—training that few nurses and physicians have received.

None of these events have contributed much, if anything, to improve the caring function of hospital staff for patients. It seems evident that caring for hospitalized patients has diminished as hospitals have responded to efforts of government and private insurers to control rapidly escalating health care costs and as medical technology and concern about diseases and patients' organs have become the dominant interest of medicine.

NURSING HOMES

As with hospitals, the modern nursing home differs greatly from institutions established in the mid-nineteenth century, which were often referred to as almshouses, poorhouses, or poor farms. By the middle of the nineteenth century, those who could not be cared for at home had few options but the almshouse (Haber, 1993). Not pleased with care in such institutions, ethnic, religious, and philanthropic organizations and individual nurses founded "homes for the aged." These homes, which typically were quite small, persisted relatively unchanged into the mid-1900s.

The present-day nursing home began to emerge with the implementation of the Hill-Burton Act in the 1950s, which encouraged the building of new and larger facilities for long-term care. Homes for the aged became nursing facilities. They were seen as an alternative to home care for the growing number of older people. In 1965, with passage of the Medicare-Medicaid legislation and the availability of funding, particularly for post-acute hospital convalescence and rehabilitation, nursing homes in the United States rapidly began to grow and change. Medicaid, for those who were medically indigent, provided funding for the "hotel costs" of nursing home care, while Medicare paid for the acute and chronic medical-care costs. As women returned to work and families were less and less able to care for sick, frail, and disabled older parents at home, placement in a nursing home became more necessary (Brody, 1990).

In 1996, there were 1.4 million residents cared for in more than 16,700 nursing homes certified by Medicaid and Medicare (Strahan, 1997). More than 82 percent of residents were aged seventy-five and older; more than one-half had one or more limitations in activities of daily living (ADLS); and more than two-thirds had limitations in instrumental activities of daily living (IADLS). Between 60 and 75 percent of all nursing home residents are thought to have a dementing illness (Kissick and Knibbe, 1989; Beck et al., 1999). With earlier discharge from hospitals, many nursing home residents who are technically classified as having subacute conditions today resemble acute-condition patients in hospitals. And, in fact, the cost of 50 percent of all new admissions to nursing homes is born by Medicare. National expenditures for nursing home care increased fivefold from 1980 to 1996, from $17.6 billion to $78.5 billion (*Statistical Abstract of the United States*, 1998).

Issues involving the quality of care in nursing homes have been a topic of deliberation for many years by federal and state governments, as well as private advocates and reformers. Licensure and regulation of facilities and assessments of operations have done little to alleviate public concern about care in most nursing homes. Concerns about care center around the fact that 67 percent of nursing homes are for-profit (Strahan, 1997) and that federal and state regulations have failed to establish adequate staffing standards in nursing homes (U.S. General Accounting Office, 1998; United Food and Commercial Workers, 1999).

Registered nurses (RNs) make up less than 7 percent of the nursing staff in nursing homes, and fewer than half of all nursing homes are required to provide twenty-four-hour RN coverage. The vast majority of care in nursing homes is delivered by certified nursing assistants, most of whom have minimal or no preparation and are paid minimum wages. Annual turnover of nursing assistants in nursing homes is 100 percent. Thus, nursing homes lack sufficient number of professional staff to meet the care and caring needs of most of their residents (Beck et al., 1999).

As few as they are, RNs are typically the only health care professionals on-site in a nursing home. Although physicians admit patients to nursing homes and are responsible for their medical care, few physicians visit their patients in nursing homes. Most nursing homes have a physician employed to oversee patient medical care, but their involvement in caring for patients is usually limited. The quality of care in nursing homes is directly dependent on the intensity of nursing care. It is well documented that caring by RNs and advanced practice geriatric nurses (geriatric nurse practitioners, clinical specialists, and gero-psychiatric clinical specialists) has positive effects on the functional status of residents, as well as other outcome measures such as resident and family satisfaction (Bleismer et al., 1998; Kayser-Jones et al., 1999; Shaughnessey et al., 1995).

HOSPICE

Perhaps the one service in which nurses have had most of the authority and responsibility for creating a climate of caring for patients is hospice. Hospice services, to provide care for patients who are terminally ill, were first developed in England then brought to the United States by nurses and clergy at Yale New Haven Nursing and Medical School and the New Haven Hospital (Moore and McCollough, 2000). Encouraged by reimbursement from Medicare, Medicaid, and some private insurers, today there are approximately three thousand hospices providing care to terminally ill patients of all ages in free-standing hospices, at home, and in hospitals and nursing homes (Mahoney, 1998).

Hospice care, provided by and supervised by professional nurses, focuses on relief of pain, symptom management, and psychological, social, and spiritual needs of patients. Families are supported during the terminal stages of a patient's illness. Unfortunately, in the United States, hospice care is not provided for many who could benefit from it in their final days. This is largely because of the attitude of many people toward dying and death as an unwelcome and even unacceptable outcome from living, as well as the attitude of some physicians that they fail if a patient dies under their care. Typically, only 20 percent of dying patients are referred to hospice, and referred patients receive a median of between seventeen and twenty-one days of hospice services prior to death (A. Jones, 1999).

Ongoing efforts to relax the six-month limit on Medicare reimbursement for hospice care and to introduce palliative care into medical and nursing practice may redress some of the antipathy of patients and physicians toward hospice. On the other hand, the "medicalization" of palliative care may serve to reduce the importance of caring activities in future hospice efforts. This is a real danger, given what has occurred when other services have been medicalized unnecessarily (e.g., obstetrical care and home care).

NURSING: A CALL TO CARING

In 1996 there were 2.56 million RNs in the United States, of whom 83 percent were employed in the profession (Moses, 1997). More than 70 percent of employed RNs work in hospitals or nursing homes (Kovner, 1998).

Nursing evolved from society's need to care for and create a caring climate for its dependent members. Before the industrial revolution, dependent family members were cared for in their homes by family members; after the industrial revolution, society had to find another method. Nursing was that method (Baer, 1998, 1999).

In the late 1800s, Florence Nightingale's work in Scutari, in the Balkans, combined with advances in public health and science and the growth of hospitals, changed the manner in which care was delivered (Nightingale, 1882). The extensive use of hospitals for the sick, the very sick, and the convalescing patient further defined the necessity for trained nurses in institutional settings. Charles Rosenberg (1987) highlighted the importance of nursing in the development of the U.S. hospital system, noting that: "Trained nurses helped impose a new social order in the wards and rooms of the hospital, and both students and trained nurses helped develop systems of care and management" (344). Lewis Thomas (1983), describing hospitals at a much later time based on his personal experience as a hospital patient, observed, "Nurses are the glue that holds the health care system together" (67).

Like patients, nurses do not differentiate between caring and care. Caring practices, "the human means for creating good outcomes" (Benner, 1999: 316), underlie the essence of nurses' work; in fact, in nursing, care itself can be the most significant contributor to cure, healing, and health. To be a good nurse requires not only technical skills but also the "ability to form helping relationships and engage in practical ethical and clinical reasoning" (Benner, 1999: 319). Thus, the notion of caring and a caring environment is not an afterthought for nurses. A call to caring is what brings people into nursing. Providing quality care and caring is what keeps people in nursing. And the inability to care eventually erodes the sense of worth that nurses have, and drives people out of nursing. To "nurse" encompasses the essential component of the nurse as a "therapeutic entity" and the nurse-patient interaction as a therapeutic relationship through which to achieve positive therapeutic goals (Peplau, 1952).

Current definitions of the nature of nursing stem from the many comments made about nursing by the discipline's founder Florence Nightingale (Nightingale, 1883). She believed that nursing was an art, requiring constant effort and education. Nightingale characterized the power of observation and attending to one's own impressions as the sine qua non of being a nurse, in that observation reveals both the facts and their meanings (Nightingale, 1882). More recently, nursing has been described as doing for patients those things they would do for themselves if they had strength, the will, and the knowledge, with the intent of promoting independence (Henderson, 1966). Orem (1971) conceptualized nursing as the promotion of "self-care" in the patient, and Peplau (1952) taught nurses to analyze the process of their interactions with patients in terms of their therapeutic quality.

While the nature of disease has changed substantially since the beginning of the century, the element of caring as integral to nursing practice has changed very little. No matter what the illness (and no matter how long or short a time a third party payer may deem hospital care necessary), patients continue to need what nurses do best: alleviate pain, calm the fearful, assist in the maintenance and restoration of health, educate and counsel patients and family members, prevent unnecessary complications and premature deaths, maintain their patients' dignity, and ease suffering at the end of life. Nursing actions are those that compensate for a person's declining (or loss of) ability to provide self-care. In collaboration with patients, families, and other health care providers, nurse assessments, decisions, and actions are wholly or partially compensatory and supportive, the priority being to reestablish quickly the patient's independence.

In 1980, the American Nurses Association offered a legal definition that reflects nursing's sense of mission about care and caring: that "nursing is the diagnosis and treatment of human responses to actual or potential health problems through such services as case finding, health, teaching, health counseling, and provision of care supportive to or restorative of life and well being" (New York State Nurses Association, 1971). Nurses' *values*—what they can and cannot do; what they should and should not do—are determined by this professional identity, as exemplified in the nurses' professional code of ethics (American Nurses Association, 1995). Nurses' *actions,* however, are tempered by the overall health care climate in which they work. They are influenced by, and at times constrained by, the expectations of patients and family members, other health care providers, health care institutions, and the laws and regulations that govern their practice. The clash between *values* and *permitted actions* is at the heart of nurses' concerns about their ability to create a climate of caring in the current health care environment.

THE CONTEMPORARY CLIMATE FOR CARING IN HOSPITALS AND NURSING HOMES

Caring, when focused on the sick, requires exquisite attention to our most basic physical and psychological needs. Caring involves intimate functions that are generally not performed for people beyond their infancy and early childhood and that, when performed for adults, usually take place within the intimacy of family. Caring draws attention to physical and psychological secrets born of vulnerability that few of us want to be reminded of once we have recovered from an illness (Fagin and Diers, 1983). We can glimpse this truth in the play *Wit,* by Edson, in which an elderly professor comforts a patient who is alone and dying of ovarian cancer by reading to her from a children's book (Edson, 1993). One must question whether the technological "assembly line" of care that currently characterizes our hospitals and nursing homes provides the subtleties and safeguards of caring that patients need and desire.

It is because the elements of caring have fallen by the wayside that patients, families, and nurses are so dissatisfied with care in hospitals and nursing homes. Today's hospitals and nursing homes are faced daily with the inherent ethical dilemma of patients being shortchanged in terms of caring. Care is under assault in even the most highly respected hospitals and nursing homes. Some observers believe that caring has been systematically destroyed by the current climate of cost reduction. Caring has never been highly valued by health care institutions, if we are to take Daniel Callahan's account in this volume (see chapter 1) at face value. Even when caring is valued and rewarded, hospital and nursing home administrators mirror society's ambivalence about the worth of caring.

All personnel who work in hospitals and nursing homes and have contact with patients could and should show concern, understanding, and kindness (the elements of caring) for patients and residents. Admission clerks, escorts, laboratory and radiology staff, secretarial or clerical and technical personnel, housekeeping staff, physical and occupational therapy staff, and others can respond to the personal needs and interests of patients. As patients undergo more diagnostic tests, procedures, and treatments, the number of hospital staff they encounter similarly increases. Each staff member can add to the patient's well-being, or conversely can add to patients feeling unperceived, unseen, uncared for. Caring for a hospitalized patient involves many different people with many different tasks and responsibilities. Interestingly, many patients will speak favorably about the attention and care they receive from personnel other than physicians, nurses, and other professionals, finding it contributes much to their well-being in the hospital.

Nevertheless, physicians and nurses have been described as key to creating what patients view as a climate of caring. As discussed in chapters 5 and 6, the life of physicians today, including the limited time they are able to spend with patients in the hospital (or in the office), makes it difficult for them to listen, learn, understand, and provide concern, compassion, empathy, and caring. As with hospitals, cost constraints and changes in the organization and delivery of medical care during recent years have further limited physicians' time with their patients. Moreover, what appears to be a movement for having "hospitalist physicians," who serve only to care for patients when hospitalized, removing patients from their usual physicians, presents further barriers to physicians knowing hospitalized patients well.

Nurses, because they are there continuously, have opportunities to understand and know patients better than do other hospital and nursing home personnel, including personal physicians. The nurse is looked to by the patient and family as the person who will guard and protect the patient from adverse experiences, and who will provide most of the patient care and caring (Louis Harris Associates, 1989, 1999).

Unfortunately, downsizing, cutbacks, and early retirement packages are systematically eliminating experienced nurses in both hospitals and nursing homes. In nursing departments, neophyte nurses now carry heavy patient loads, perform complex technical tasks, and supervise unprepared, nonprofessional nursing personnel; they are not given the oversight of experienced nurses deemed so essential by Nightingale and others. The "contemporary" administrative techniques of cross-training, assigning nurses to various units in various specialties, and the phenomenon of "just in time" nursing, where nurses are called in and let go on the basis of daily shifts in patient census, further underscores the lack of understanding of the essential element of caring and the sustained relationships that underpin caring environments. Moreover, nursing staff are now heavily involved in administrative work such as record keeping and managing other personnel—activities that absorb time that should be available to meet patients' personal needs.

Strangely, in a financial climate that rewards short stays in hospital and lowered readmission rates, close attention to patient care and to caring should matter to administrators. The limited time that nurses have for face-to-face conversations and education leaves patients and families ill-equipped to provide care at home. With patients who are dying and those with complex and rapidly changing drug and treatment regimens (i.e., patients with predominantly multiple and chronic health conditions), knowing the patient and the patient's concerns is the best vehicle to avoid untoward patient events. Yet this monitoring is increasingly devalued in hospitals and nursing homes: direct patient contact is moved down to nonprofessional providers, and the professional providers—nurses, physicians and social workers—have limitations placed on their having direct contacts with patients. Through such inattention to the caring aspects of care, increasingly the condition of a patient worsens after discharge and the patient has then to be readmitted to hospital (Kovner, 1998).

NURSES AND THE ETHICAL DILEMMAS OF CARING

The ethical dilemmas that nurses face today in promoting caring are both different and the same as those they faced decades ago. Fulfilling the public trust that they "do no harm" is a matter of daily concern of health care professionals, as it has always been. Yet the added wrinkle of the market has created new barriers that impede the ability of nurses and others to move forward an agenda of caring in hospitals and nursing homes. In a market-driven environment, nurses increasingly find that the multiple and often competing mandates of medical research, treatment, and cost make it more and more difficult to keep the patient their primary concern, making the fulfillment of patients' needs for caring more difficult and profound.

Below we discuss three types of ethical dilemmas that serve to illustrate the conflicts nurses face in fulfilling their mandate to create a caring environment in hospitals and nursing homes.

Providing Care in an Unsafe Environment

One of the fundamental ethical dilemmas facing nurses lies in having to choose which of two approaches least violates their obligation to care for a patient. The choices are between (1) refusing to work and (2) continuing to work in an environment that precludes caring—for example, where there is short-staffing, poorly prepared staff, inadequate medical backup—and refusing requests to do procedures or treatments for which the nurse is unprepared or poorly prepared, thus having no time to provide compassionate care.

Nurses' professional code of ethics requires that they never abandon a patient. Nurses are taught that no matter what the circumstances, their job is to stay in the situation and provide care. In Beth Norman's book about the ninety-five U.S. Army and Navy nurses who were imprisoned in the Philippines for more than three years during World War II, the saddest moment the nurses remember from the war was being ordered to abandon soldiers in jungle hospitals to certain Japanese capture (Norman, 1999). Reluctance to abandon the patient is what keeps nurses at the bedside long after their shifts are finished and what drives them to work double shifts in hospitals and nursing homes.

But leaving the bedside is not the only form of patient abandonment. Because people place such great trust in nurses, their continued presence in an unsafe situation also constitutes a form of patient abandonment. A nurse at the bedside creates a sense of safety for patients. Nurses represent a hospital's "*Good Housekeeping* Seal of Approval." Because they are seen by the public as "caring professionals" (Louis Harris Associates, 1989,

1999), patients trust nurses to recognize and act when they are taking a turn for the worse, to know when technology is or is not working, and to head off untoward events. When nurses remain at the bedside, the patient should have reason to feel secure—that all is well, that a professional cares.

In this age of high technology, care of patients is complex and involves multiple treatments. On any given day, patients in intensive care units receive an average of 178 different interventions (Leape, 1995). When nurse staffing is insufficient and when nurses do not "know" the patient, patients suffer injuries and infections: they receive late medications, treatments, and meals (or entirely miss them); they have complications that are not picked up early, such as blood clots and urinary-tract infections; and they fail to receive caring that promotes healing and recovery. Thus, when nurses continue to provide care in situations they know to be uncaring and unsafe, patients may be unaware that they have been placed at risk for untoward events.

The dilemma is compounded because nurses who raise issues of poor care and lack of caring often are accused of being "self serving"; they also risk losing their jobs (*New York Times,* 1999). Thus, nurses constantly face the conflict involved in continuing to provide care in a fashion that they know places patients at risk.

Inadequate Power to Create a Caring Environment

A hallmark of a profession is the power to control the terms, conditions, and contents of work. Although nurses are educated as professionals to act in accordance with professional criteria, they quickly become frustrated and disillusioned when they enter a work setting that prohibits them from exercising and fulfilling their rights and responsibilities to care. Many nurses are critical of other nurses who fail to take caring responsibilities seriously. In fact, nurses are often critical of one another instead of offering each other the support necessary to more correctly identify power discrepancies that limit their authority to care.

In hospitals and nursing homes, when nurses lose their accountability they lose their ability to influence the care environment. This is what is happening in many hospitals and nursing homes today. As noted above, hospitals have taken steps that alarmingly denigrate the nursing ethic of caring, advocacy, and accountability by downsizing and use of unlicensed personnel to substitute for professional nurses. Perhaps most dramatically, in an attempt to mirror the market strategy of "product line," many hospitals have eliminated nursing departments altogether, making nursing virtually invisible within the hospital organization structure (Fulmer, 1999). In a health care system in which nursing has been made invisible, who will stand up for the patient's need for caring?

The Mislabeling of Medical Errors: Blaming the Provider, Not the System

Untoward events that happen in hospitals and nursing homes are of increasing concern to patients and providers. Many of these untoward events are blamed on individual errors made by nurses and doctors; in fact, the majority of these errors stem from system flaws within the health care setting. This is particularly evident in nursing homes, where unprepared, understaffed, and unsupervised nonlicensed staff are often called on to provide care beyond their scope of practice in an environment where profit motives openly conflict with quality-of-care goals.

Through such identification of nurses and physicians as the cause of errors, patients are encouraged to think of these health care providers as "uncaring." Thus, inaccurate labeling of medical errors—calling them provider failures rather than system failures—undermines the public trust in health care professionals. Properly designed systems and safeguards can help address many of the lapses in care. "Human beings make mistakes because the systems, tasks and processes they work in are poorly designed and poorly executed" (Leape, 1995: 39). Examples of dilemmas and errors that need system solutions rather than individual-provider solutions are numerous. They are evident in the errors that occur when a nurse is ordered to rotate to a pediatric unit that is short-staffed but where the rotating nurse knows that her lack of pediatric experience makes her unfit to provide care on that unit. They are evident in the falls and delirium that occur in severely functionally and mentally incapacitated residents who are inappropriately and uncaringly transferred from nursing homes to the hospital. And they are evident in the physical injuries and psychological scars that result from the use of physical restraints by staff working in environments that limit human contact and individualized care: more contact and care would reduce the need for the use of patient restraints. Failure to redress system errors stifles nurses' willingness to identify potential sources of error, limits nurses' ability to care, and continues to place patients at risk.

TOWARD THE IMPROVEMENT OF CARING IN INSTITUTIONAL SETTINGS

Reestablishing the centrality of caring in health care institutions cannot be achieved easily in a medical environment where, as Callahan (chapter 1) puts it, "caring, as a value, can be downgraded, delisted, maybe someday eliminated." But if we listen to the anguish of health care consumers and practicing nurses and physicians, the absence of a sense of caring threatens our whole health care system and our ability to continue to attract the best and the brightest to the helping professions.

Hospitals and nursing homes have become fragile institutions. Subject to complex diagnostic and treatment options within a system pervaded by cost cutters and the high-tech/science medical system, patients have never had a greater need for caring. An increasingly vulnerable patient population—that admitted during the most acute or needy part of the health-to-illness trajectory—is dramatically dependent on nursing care (Louis Harris Associates, 1999). Patients are fearful that a nurse will not be there when needed, and family members are often quoted as saying, "If I had not been with my relative or friend, she might have died or not received the care she needed."

Continued financial cutbacks in hospital staffing ignore data showing that restructuring has failed to achieve desired cost reductions and has reduced the patient's sense of being cared for. On the other hand, a growing body of research confirms what consumers have long known: that there is a significant positive relationship between the presence of professional nurses and patients feeling satisfied with their care and other patient outcomes—such as the avoidance of hospital-acquired infections, bedsores, medication errors, patient falls, and urinary-tract infections (Aiken, 1994; Kovner, 1998). Study after study confirms that higher nurse/patient ratios, organizations responsive to nurse autonomy, and positive relations between nurses and physicians lower mortality and morbidity and improve care and caregiving in hospitals and nursing homes. Research on failure to resuscitate, defined as the death of a patient after a complication, links nurse staffing as the variable most related to patient outcomes (Silber and Rosenbaum, 1997). These findings should not be a surprise since clinical grasp and clinical forethought, the hallmarks of professional nursing (Benner, 1999), are essential to the first steps of rescue: identification and surveillance—that is, "knowing" the patient.

It is crucial for the future of caring that the dilemmas nurses face—

providing care in an unsafe environment, inadequate power to create a caring environment, and the mislabeling of medical errors as provider failures rather than system failures—be dealt with now and not later as hospitals and nursing homes begin the twenty-first century. Most bedside nurses today do not see themselves as leaders or as powerful people; rather, they say that they are unsupported and unable to appropriately care for patients. They report stress and frustration and feel that they receive little recognition for what they do. Although the public trusts and respects nurses more than all other health professionals (Louis Harris Associates, 1989, 1999), this respect is not transferred into support and recognition for the bedside nurse by hospitals and nursing homes. Health care institutions need a vision that values care and the caregivers charged with assuring a caring environment.

Hospitals and nursing homes might expand the mandates of their ethics committees so that they can become platforms for discussion of the ethical dilemmas of caring in the institution. If they applied mediation techniques and procedures (Dubler, 1994), these interdisciplinary committees could provide the vehicle for nurses, physicians, administrators, and others to discuss and resolve issues that may initially appear divisive but just as often can be reframed as unifying issues among disciplines. Without a structural and procedural mechanism for examining and resolving issues of caring, institutions will remain mired in the kind of situations described in this chapter. This is especially true in nursing homes, but it is also true in hospitals. The examples we cite are characteristic of situations that will increasingly confront us if we do not turn our attention to the caring of patients. No set of issues can be more challenging. No set of issues can be more crucial.

REFERENCES

Aiken, L. (1994). Lower Medicare mortality among a set of hospitals known for nursing care. *Medical Care* 32(8): 771–78.

American Hospital Association (AHA) (1997). *Eye on Patients.* Chicago, IL: AHA.

American Hospital Association (1999). *Hospital Statistics.* Chicago, IL: AHA.

American Nurses Association (ANA) (1995). *Code for Nurses.* Washington, DC: ANA.

Baer, E. (1998). The philosophical and historical bases of advanced practice nursing roles. In M. Mezey and D. O. McGivern, eds., *Nurses, Nurse Practitioners: Evolution to Advanced Practice,* 3rd ed., pp. 72-91. New York: Springer Publishing.

Baer, E. (1999). Untitled paper prepared for the Milbank Memorial Fund, New York.

Beck, C., Ortigara, A., Mercer, S., and Shue, V. (1999). Enabling and empowering certified nursing assistants for quality dementia care. *International Journal of Geriatric Psychiatry* 14(3): 197–221.

Benner, P. (1999). Claiming the wisdom and worth of clinical practice. *Nursing and Health Care Perspectives* 20(6): 312–19.

Bleismer, M. M., Smayling, M., Kane, R., and Shannon, I. (1998). The relationship between nursing staffing levels and nursing home outcomes. *Journal of Aging and Health* 10: 351–71.

Brody, E. (1990). *Women in the Middle: Their Parent-Care Years.* New York: Springer Publishing.

Dubler, N. (1994). *Mediating Bioethical Disputes.* New York: United Hospital Fund.

Edson, M. (1993). *Wit.* New York: Faber & Faber.

Fagin, C., and Diers, D. (1983). Nursing as a metaphor. *New England Journal of Medicine* 309: 116–17.

Fulmer, T. (1999). Personal communication to Mathy Mezey. Division of Nursing, New York University.

Haber, C. (1993). Over the hill to the poorhouse: Rhetoric and reality in the institutional history of the aged. In K. W. Schaie and W. A. Achenbaum, eds., *Societal Impact on Aging: Historical Perspectives,* pp. 90–113. New York: Springer Publishing.

Henderson, V. (1966) *The Nature of Nursing.* New York: Macmillan.

Jones, A. (1999). Personal communication to Mathy Mezey from the president and CEO of the New York State Hospice Association, October 12.

Kayser-Jones, J., Schell, E. S., Porter, C., Barbaccia, J. U. C., and Shaw, H. (1999). Factors contributing to dehydration in nursing homes: Inadequate staffing and lack of professional supervision. *Journal of the American Geriatric Society,* 47: 1187–94.

Kissick, W. L., and Knibbe, K. K. (1989). Patient's needs, societal resources, and nursing strategies. In M. D. Mezey, J. E. Lynaugh, and M. M. Cartier, eds., *Nursing Homes and Nursing Care: Lessons from the Teaching Nursing Homes,* pp. 12–29. New York: Springer Publishing.

Kovner, C. (1998). Nurse staffing levels and adverse events following surgery in U.S. hospitals. *Image* 30(4): 315–21.

Leape, M. (1995). Systems analysis of adverse drug events. *Journal of the American Medical Association.* 274: 35–43.

Louis Harris Associates (1989). *Poll on Nurses and Health Care.* New York: National League for Nursing.

Louis Harris Associates (1999). Poll prepared for Sigma Theta Tau International and NurseWeek Publishing, www.nursingsociety.org/media/exec_smry_hrs-poll.html.

Mahoney, J. (1998). The Medicare hospice benefit—15 years of success. *Journal of Palliative Medicine* 1(2): 139–46.

Moore, P. C., and McCollough, R. H. (2000). Hospice: End-of-life care at home.

In R. H. Binstock and L. E. Cluff, eds., *Home Care Advances: Essential Research and Policy Issues,* pp. 101–16. New York: Springer Publishing.

Moses, E. B. (1997). *The Registered Nurse Population: Findings from the National Sample Survey of Registered Nurses, March 1996.* Washington, DC: U.S. Department of Health and Human Services, Health Resources and Services Administration, Division of Nursing, September.

New York State Nurses Association (NYSNA) (1971). *Title and Education Law, Article 139, Part 6902.* New York: NYSNA.

New York Times (1999). Tentative deal averts strike by nurses. August 10.

Nightingale, E. F. (1882). Training of nurses and nursing the sick [s.v., Nurses, training of]. In *Quains Dictionary of Medicine.* London: Privately printed.

Nightingale, E. F. (1883). *Address to the Probationer Nurses in the Nightingale Fund School.* London: Spottiswoode.

Norman, E. (1999). *We Band of Angels.* New York: Random House.

Orem, D. (1971). *Nursing: Concepts of Practice.* New York: McGraw-Hill.

Peplau, H. (1952). *Interpersonal Relations in Nursing.* New York: Putnam.

Risse, G. B. (1999). *Mending Bodies, Saving Souls: A History of Hospitals.* Oxford: Oxford University Press.

Rosenberg, C. (1987). *The Care of Strangers.* New York: Basic Books.

Shaughnessey, P. L., Kramer, A., Hittle, D., and Steiner, J. (1995). Quality of care in teaching nursing homes: Findings and implications. *Health Care Financing Review* 16(4): 55–82.

Shryock, R. H. (1936). *The Development of Modern Medicine: An Interpretation of the Social and Scientific Factors Involved.* Philadelphia: University of Pennsylvania Press.

Silber, J. H., and Rosenbaum, P. R. (1997). A spurious correlation between hospital mortality and complication rates. *Medical Care* 35(10): 77–92.

Statistical Abstract of the United States (1998). Washington, DC: U.S. Department of Commerce, Bureau of the Census.

Strahan, G. (1997). *An Overview of Nursing Homes and Their Current Residents: Data from the 1995 National Nursing Home Survey.* Advance Data #280. Centers for Disease Control and Prevention / National Center for Health Statistics, Vital and Health Statistics.

Thomas, L. (1983). *The Youngest Science: Notes of a Medicine Watcher.* New York: Viking Press.

United Food and Commercial Workers (1999). *The Care Gap: A Report on Patient Care and Profits at Beverly Enterprises Inc. in Alabama.* Washington, DC: United Food and Commercial Workers.

U.S. General Accounting Office (1998). *California Nursing Homes: Care Problems Persist Despite Federal and State Oversight.* Report to the Special Committee on Aging, U.S. Senate. GAO/HEHS-98-202. Washington, DC: U.S. Government Printing Office.

8

Home- and Community-Based Care
Toward a Caring Paradigm

ROBYN I. STONE, DR.P.H.

HOME- and community-based care (HCBC) is not a new phenomenon on the frontier of caring; rather, it is one of the "early pioneers." Families and friends in the community have been caring for disabled and chronically or acutely ill individuals for centuries. In the last third of the twentieth century, public reimbursement supported a tremendous expansion of nursing homes in the United States through the Medicaid program (for long-term care) and the Medicare program (for subacute care and rehabilitation). Yet most Americans still have a strong attachment to the intrinsic value of "home," combined with an intense animosity toward institutionalization.

"I would rather die than be forced to live in a nursing home!" This is the mantra of millions of the elderly, as well as younger, disabled, people, who fear that their current or future needs for care will result in institutionalization. Families also express this concern and are determined to avoid this option, if at all possible. In fact, among people with disabling conditions, the vast majority—95 percent of those under sixty-five years old and 72 percent of those aged sixty-five and older—receive long-term care in their own homes or in community-based settings (Komisar, Lambrew, and Feder, 1996). Most of this care is provided in the home "free" by family members, friends, and others, an army of *informal* caregivers who help to maintain the home as the primary setting for caring for persons who need long-term care and a major setting for those who require subacute care and rehabilitation.

Several factors unique to the latter part of the twentieth century, however, have contributed to the professionalization of HCBC. The aging of the population, the survival and extended longevity of people born with or experiencing significant disabilities prior to old age, and the increase in women's participation in the labor force, have converged to place new and competing demands on what had been predominantly an informal system of care. Moreover, a steadfast belief by public officials in the cost effectiveness of noninstitutional long-term care settings (despite evidence to the contrary), has led to a shift toward *formal,* paid, HCBC options that are financed through public programs and private-sector developments. For example, while total Medicaid long-term care spending increased 9.9 percent between 1988 and 1998, the spending for home- and community-based programs funded through special Medicaid waivers granted to state governments increased 30.5 percent (Burwell, 1999). Medicare home health expenditures grew exponentially between 1988 and 1996, by 762 percent (Binstock and Cluff, 2000), leading Congress to enact significant cuts in this benefit in the Balanced Budget Act of 1997.

In our enthusiasm to help maintain disabled and chronically ill people in the community, as formal, paid, professionalized care increases, we must understand the tradeoffs and potentially negative consequences for individuals and their families. Has caring, an important element of caregiving, gotten lost in our preoccupation with the formal, technical aspects of providing care? And even when families and other informal caregivers are central in providing care, are there factors that inhibit the quantity and quality of caring that can take place?

Sociologists and ethicists have explored the differences between *care* and *caring,* uncovering the bold truth that home care and family care are not synonymous with caring. Tronto (1998: 16) defines care as "a species activity that includes everything that we do to maintain, continue, and repair our 'world' so that we can live in it as well as possible. The world includes our bodies, our selves, and our environment, all of which we seek to interweave in a complex, life-sustaining web." From an instrumental perspective, care does not require caring; it simply involves performing the tasks required to meet some goal. Caring, however, has an important relational aspect that focuses on the human interaction between the caregiver and the care recipient. Baines, Evans, and Neysmith (1991: 11) define caring as "the mental, emotional and physical efforts involved in looking after, responding to, and supporting others."

This chapter considers caring within the magnitude and scope of home- and community-based care in the United States today and highlights key issues that have emerged in our zeal to provide care in home and community settings. It begins with a brief overview of the definitions of home, home care, and community-based care, followed by a discussion of the role of "caring" in HCBC. Barriers to caring are then discussed, focusing on issues in both the informal and formal care sectors. Next, two important emerging trends in HCBC—*assisted living* and *consumer direction*—are reviewed with an emphasis on the potential for caring in these models. The chapter concludes with a discussion of how a more balanced view of HCBC, which encourages and rewards caring as well as the tasks of care, may help to shape the nature of financing, delivering, and preparing a workforce to provide appropriate care that includes caring.

THE MEANING OF *HOME*

Home care is viewed by many as a "paradigm of choice" because it allows people to stay at home, protecting them from coercion and the constraints of institutionalization (Collopy, Dubler, and Zuckerman, 1990). While the nursing home evokes images of abandonment and family failures, home care promises independence and social integration, enabling individuals to remain in a familiar and comfortable environment in which they can maximize control over their lives. The home is private territory—the occupant's own personal space. At home, one has, at least in theory, a degree of power that is not evidenced in a hospital or nursing home (Twigg, 1997). In addition to privacy, home is also associated with ease, a haven from the sometimes harsh outside world (Sixsmith, 1990).

The concept of home expresses love, unity, and caring, and is believed by many to have a restorative effect beyond the technical aspects of caregiving. Home is more than a passive setting in which caregiving happens to take place just because it is easier or because a family member may feel a responsibility. Rather, home "represents both a cultural (shared) system for order and each person's interpretation or version of shared community values about space, organization, and being" (Rubinstein, 1990: 38). The objects of home can provide links to the past; who a person is and has been can be expressed in that person's surroundings and in the deployment of possessions in them. For many, each room in the house may have special meaning—the dining room where the family gathers; the special reading nook, television room, or screened-in porch where private moments were spent. Furthermore, there is meaning in keeping a person "at home" rather than in a hospital or nursing home: it can mean that the person is not fully sick or incapacitated.

In the ideal, home care occupies a morally and socially unassailable position (Bayer, 1986). But, as will be highlighted later in this chapter, the realities of providing care in the home, a setting not naturally designed for many of the required activities, are often in conflict with the warm and comforting images of home and the ideal of caring.

DEFINING HOME- AND COMMUNITY-BASED CARE

Home- and community-based care is a catchall phrase that refers to a wide variety of noninstitutional settings in which care is provided. These settings range from the private home of the individual or the family to community-based residential facilities—congregate living arrangements in which various levels and types of day services are available. The majority of people with disabilities and chronic illness receive care at home, either in their own home or in the home of a close relative or friend.

Much of the gerontological literature refers to a continuum of care, identifying the nursing home as the most restrictive setting and one's own home as the least restrictive. Kane, Kane, and Ladd (1998) and I (Stone, 2000) have challenged this linear concept, suggesting that instead a repertoire of services and settings should be available at any one point in time, and across time and place, to meet the needs, preferences, and circumstances of an individual and family. Furthermore, in the description of a continuum mentioned above, the term *least restrictive* is somewhat illusory since a homebound elder may have less autonomy than another person living in a nursing home or residential setting.

Care services encompass a broad range of assistance with the daily activities of living: such assistance (as well as medical care) is needed by chronically ill and disabled individuals over a prolonged period of time. For those needing long-term care, the services are primarily low-tech, designed to minimize, rehabilitate, or compensate for loss of independent physical or mental functioning due to an underlying condition or disability. These services include hands-on and standby or supervisory assistance as well as the use of assistive devices such as canes and walkers, and technology such as computerized medication reminders and emergency alert systems. HCBC may also include modifications to the home, such as the building of ramps and the installation of grab bars in bathrooms and disability-friendly door handles on doors and cabinets. For younger, working-age people with disabilities, personal-care attendants and assistive devices may be the essential HCBC elements; such assistance can help individuals obtain and retain employment.

As federal and state policies have provided financial incentives to discharge patients quickly from hospitals (or to bypass hospitals entirely), medically oriented acute, postacute, and rehabilitative care has been increasingly provided in home- and community-based settings. For postacute (typically posthospital) care needs, individuals may receive skilled nursing and high-tech services in the home, including intravenous drug therapy, ventilator assistance, and wound care. This care is generally short-term and geared toward rehabilitation and restoration. In addition, the majority of terminally ill persons who opt for hospice services are cared for in the home (Moore and McCollough, 2000). Hospice care focuses on caring and palliation of pain.

In many communities, adult day care programs have been established to meet the needs of a primarily elderly long-term care population. According to the National Adult Day Services Association (1999), these centers are designed to serve adults who are physically impaired or mentally confused and may require supervision, increased social opportunities, assistance with personal care, or other daily living activities. The average age of the adult day services consumer is seventy-six, and two-thirds are women. It is estimated that in the United States more than four thousand adult day centers are currently serving approximately two hundred thousand disabled and chronically ill people and their families; most are nonprofit and many are affiliated with larger organizations such as home care agencies, skilled nursing facilities, or multipurpose senior organizations.

The most common form of adult day care is a social model in which relatively disabled elders receive ongoing supervision and personal care, as well as social integration and companionship, in a group setting. The hours usually parallel the five-day, nine-to-five workweek, with a limited number of programs operating on the weekends; only a fraction experiment with evening and night hours. Transportation to and from the site may be provided as part of the purchased package of services (services are publicly subsidized for low-income participants). Some programs primarily serve a clientele that is physically disabled; others target the cognitively impaired, with special interventions for people with Alzheimer disease and other dementias.

A less common, and more intensive, form of adult day care is the day health model. This option provides medical primary care, case management, and long-term care services in community settings to severely disabled elders who live in a private home or in congregate housing. Perhaps the best-known example of a community-based intervention built around the adult day health model is the Program of All-Inclusive Care for the Elderly (PACE), a fully capitated health and long-term care delivery system for disabled, nursing-home-certifiable individuals, funded by Medicaid and Medicare (see Branch, Coulam, and Zimmerman, 1995).

Adult day care is not a preferred modality for all disabled and chronically ill older persons living in the community; nor is it appropriate for everyone. But where it does work, it provides an important source of respite for primary informal caregivers, as well as services, social interaction, and supervision of the care recipient. It allows caregivers (who may, for example, have paid employment responsibilities) to attend to other important parts of their lives—as well as giving them a well-deserved break from caregiving obligations.

Residential care is an ambiguous category of home- and community-based care that includes such settings as board-and-care, adult foster care homes, and assisted living. (Some refer to board-and-care as the "poor person's assisted living" because the occupants are low-income, and room and board are often subsidized by federal and state Supplemental Security Income [SSI] payments.) The licensing and regulation of residential care varies by state and locality; consequently, there is no consensus on the definition of residential care or nationwide estimate of the number of such facilities. Nomenclature, size of facility, and magnitude and scope of the services vary tremendously (Newcomer and Stone, 1985; Mollica, 1998). One recent study of assisted living (Hawes, Rose, and Phillips, 1999) reported, as of early 1998, an estimated 11,472 facilities with approximately 558,400 residents. (The definition of assisted living in this study covered facilities with eleven or more beds that served a primarily elderly population, providing twenty-four-hour oversight, housekeeping, and at least two meals a day; there also had to be personal assistance with at least two of the following three activities: taking medications, bathing, and dressing.)

Residential care tends to be viewed conceptually as an option for individuals who may not require assistance at nursing home level but who are no longer able to remain in their own homes or with a family member. It is thus seen primarily as a substitute for living at home and, for some, a step in a downward trajectory toward placement in a nursing home. However, some states (e.g., Oregon) have been aggressively using residential care alternatives as substitutes for nursing homes, with substantial numbers of very disabled individuals being relocated to assisted-living or adult foster homes.

THE ROLE OF CARING IN CARE

In each of the HCBC settings described above, "caring for" and "caring about" the individual should be coequal. Compassion, comfort, and communication are as important as the provision of skilled care or help with bathing, dressing, and eating. Trust and rapport between caregiver and care recipient are essential elements.

The importance of the relational aspect of care was highlighted in the findings of a study of home care clients and their workers (Eustis and Fischer, 1991). The most frequent client complaints were not about job performance but about the quality of the interpersonal dynamics with their workers, particularly poor communication and a lack of sensitivity. Home care workers live with an undercurrent of tension between their clients' desires for company and companionship and the more instrumental care they are trained and paid to provide (Stone, 1999). Human relationships may be jeopardized when care is reduced to instrumental tasks and individuals are judged by task performance only.

In her work on the ethic of care, Noddings (1984, 1995) distinguishes between "natural caring," which is driven by love or inclination, and "ethical caring," which has to be summoned by obedience to duty; the latter arises out of memories of caring and being cared for and the valuation placed on caring by the caregiver. Noddings argues that ethical caring cannot supplant natural caring and that the emphasis in home care should be on moral support rather than obligation, on caring and relation rather than on an abstract ethical principle and individual moral authority.

Some feminist writers who have examined the "labor of caregiving" criticize the concept of natural or intrinsic caregiving for its role in fostering powerlessness among women, arguing that questions about care's intrinsic value are not only naive but pernicious (Abel, 1991; Clement, 1996). Others have suggested that acknowledging the labor involved in caregiving, not just the caring aspects but the work involved, is essential to achieving better benefits and perhaps more parity with men, who have not been the primary caregivers. Nevertheless, care is an expression of identity, whereas work may be viewed as a mere transaction of goods and services. From this perspective, care is degraded if referred to as work (Clement, 1996).

Brown and Stetz (1999) have developed a model of family caregiving at home for a relative with a potentially fatal illness. They identify several stages of caregiving, including the initial phase of "choosing to care," which is motivated by both a sense of obligation and reciprocity, and "taking care," which involves guiding, giving, and doing for the person to meet the individual's needs—managing the illness, struggling with the health care system, and managing the environment as well as dealing with one's own personal suffering, responding to family issues, and preparing for the death.

MacRae (1998) points out that caring involves an ongoing series of interaction situations that must be defined and negotiated. For family caregivers, defining and negotiating situations are complex; negotiation is an ongoing intimate activity and often involves a complicated relationship with a significant other. MacRae suggests that caring is "emotional work" that often requires managing one's own emotions as well as the care recipient's inability to control emotions. Clement (1996) warns, however, that definitions of care should not be limited or reducible to feelings; the acknowledgment of care as work—both the physical tasks and the feelings management—explicitly recognizes the social importance of this role.

It is also important to point out that for some people with physical disabilities, the provision of hands-on personal care by professionals in the home is not perceived as "caring"; rather, it is seen as a violation of their personal boundaries and a serious invasion of their untouchable zones. In one study of disabled individuals, Lillesto (1997) found that many of them feel that their caregivers treat them as objects, leading to a strong sense of depersonalization. As one respondent commented: "She as a person is no longer there, only her body, constantly reminding her of her weaknesses and what she cannot do" (289). To compensate, many care recipients consider their bodies "public" when professional caregivers are in the home; they themselves depersonalize their bodies in order to cope with the violation.

BARRIERS TO CARING IN HCBC

While home- and community-based options are viscerally appealing to the vast majority of people who are faced with care decisions, it is important to understand the limitations of HCBC as "caring" alternatives to institutionalization. Private homes have not usually been designed around the needs and limitations of a care recipient; in fact, the physical environment of a private home can actually impede an individual's performance of the activities of daily living (ADLs): stairways, poorly lit hallways, and scatter rugs can make it increasingly difficult for people with disabilities and chronic illnesses to live independently (Aulisio, May, and Aulisio, 1998). The introduction of high-tech care into the home also poses special physical and emotional challenges to the individual and family. Finding adequate space for equipment is but one issue. Turning the dining room or living room, where the family has gathered for years, into a "sick room" can destroy the meaning of these living spaces for those who remain there. As Arras and Dubler (1995) note: "Rooms occupied by the paraphernalia of high-tech medicine may cease to be what they once were in the minds of their occupants; familiar and comforting family rituals, such as holiday meals, may lose their charm when continued around a mammoth flexi-care bed, and much of the privacy and intimacy of ordinary family life may be sacrificed to the institutional culture that trails in the wake of high-tech medicine" (3).

The home is more than a physical place: it represents a sense of "domestic order" that involves both the use of space and the role of routines and procedures in daily life (Rubinstein, 1990: 41). The introduction of home care changes that order. For those who see home as a haven or refuge, the care of a disabled or chronically ill family member, particularly a demented parent, can cause significant disorder. For those who define home as the aggregate of life events and routines representing personal development, the home may be "put on hold."

Limitations on Caring in Informal Care

Although family members—wives and daughters, in particular—provide most long-term care in the United States, family caring should not be idealized or romanticized. Family caregiving is often filled with conflict and tension, even under the best of circumstances. Abel's (1991) study of adult daughters caring for disabled parents found that many caregivers, reciprocating care they had received as children, expressed concern about demeaning the parent. It is very difficult for a mother or father to be cared for *like* a child *by* a child; and such caring is even more heartwrenching for the adult children.

The literature on elder abuse underscores the facts that the quality of caring in family care may be problematic and that informal home care is not always the best option (Quinn and Tomita, 1997). Recurrent cases of abuse and neglect by the family caregiver may not be intentional but may be due to stress, ignorance, apathy, or the caregiver's own frailty and advanced age. In many situations, long-standing conflicts and estrangements between family members are exacerbated when a child or spouse is then "forced" into a caregiving role out of obligation or financial necessity. Some family members care for elders or younger disabled relatives because of their own pathology and inability to avail themselves of other supports. Brody (1985) referred to "excessive caregiving" among adult children who are in the fruitless search for parental affection and approval. Such caregivers may continue to care for an elderly parent even when the physical and emotional care needs of the recipient indicate that institutional placement would benefit the individual and the family.

The introduction of high-tech interventions in the home is placing significant responsibilities on family members with neither the training nor the basic capacity to perform such duties. Arras and Dubler (1995) have lamented that even when there is a real possibility of the individual remaining in the hospital or nursing home, the choice between the institution and home may be illusory. There is, for example, no real choice for a mother who is asked whether she would prefer her ventilator-dependent child to go home or remain in a hospital or nursing home. To say no would be to commit the child to an institution, a decision that would lead many to label the mother a bad and uncaring parent.

Similarly, some informal caregivers become secondary victims of such conditions as Alzheimer disease (Kuhn, 1998). The heroic decision to continue to provide home care to a combative, disruptive parent or spouse with dementia can be an emotionally and physically dangerous option for the caregiver as well as the care recipient. But the moral blame (real or perceived) associated with institutionalizing a loved one discourages many families from making an unpleasant but more appropriate placement decision.

Caring and the Professionalization of HCBC

Many researchers and long-term care analysts who have explored the effects of professionalization and "bureaucratization" of home care and other community-based services (see, for example, Collopy, Dubler, and Zuckerman, 1990; Clement, 1996; Stone, 1999) agree that there is a "clash between the norms of caring in private relationships and the norms of efficiency, professionalism and accountability in business and government" (Stone, 1999: 61). When care is recast as an economic and bureaucratic good, deep norms about compassion, altruism, generosity, and cooperation are reshaped as well. Most ordinary people caring for family members do not think about progressing toward goals; they think about their relationships and how to best meet the needs of the disabled child, spouse, or parent. However, when judgment and compassion come under public scrutiny, the accountability brings moral confusion to the world of care.

The situation is especially problematic for the home health care aide or personal care worker—the frontline caregiver who provides the majority of hands-on assistance to the disabled individual. In their description of the culture of home health aides, Glasser and Brecker (1997) note that the human dimension of the work is essential, that the caring role is embedded in the tradition of the home care worker. The home care system, however, is thick with institutional structures and controls that often undermine the norms of caring. There are significant disparities between what home health aides are allowed to do as certified and licensed paraprofessionals (as strangers) and what they are allowed to do as ordinary citizens, relatives, or friends. Agencies strongly advise against "getting too emotionally attached," although that is one of the tenets of a "caring" paradigm. Even though home care workers recognize the importance of emotional and relational activities that help them to get their instrumental tasks done, they describe this "caring" work as "outside the job" or "nonwork" (Aronson and Neysmith, 1996).

Caregivers talk about their personal attachments to their clients as though their deep affection, loyalty, and overflowing generosity were somehow illicit (Stone, 1999). Recognizing that good care often requires attention to the spouse and other family members of their clients, many home health aides visit the care recipients on their days off. This allows them to engage in some of the more personal activities not allowed or rewarded by agencies and also offers respite to the family. Workers have to justify their personal relationships with their clients as "being a friend" so that they will not be accused of breaking government or agency rules.

The bureaucratization of care creates a real paradox for the home care worker. On the one hand, the caregiver's personal relationship to the client allows the worker to know the individual as a person rather than an abstraction. The expertise that the caregiver gains through this close contact, however, is not recognized by the system. In fact, the generalist who is at a distance (the supervising nurse or physician) is considered the expert in caring, and the personal contact in care work must be monitored by the professional. The closer the worker is to the client, therefore, the less likely it is that the worker is allowed autonomy. Since care work is defined by the bureaucracy as taking "good instructions" from others, the frontline worker may be prohibited from doing what she or he believes should be done for the client out of moral commitment to another human being. To be an autonomous worker, one must be professional; but to be a professional, one must shed personalized caregiving tasks. Because administration of prescription drugs is generally prohibited, the worker is not allowed to rub a prescription cream on the back of a client—even a client who cannot reach there. Due to liability concerns, the worker is also not allowed to lift a care recipient who falls to the floor. The shift in priorities from caring to clearly defined instrumental tasks perpetuates itself. The requirement that caregivers focus their energies on quantifiable activities that are free of risk results in high turnover rates among caregivers, which in turn hinders the development of the personal relationships essential to more holistic care.

Some states have shown some sensitivity to this dilemma, moderating their legislation governing "nurse practice" to allow delegation of certain tasks such as medication administration, wound care, and the changing of catheters to home care aides (Kane, 1997). For workers who have developed (or may develop) an intimate relationship with their clients, these functions are as important and must be done with as much sensitivity as bathing, dressing, and toileting. A number of states (Oregon, Kansas, Texas, Minnesota, New York) have included provisions for nurse delegation, but the latitude and interpretations vary tremendously. These initiatives have met with serious resistance by many of the nurses' organizations, and the professional turf issues are as significant as the care issues. The battle over nurse delegation exemplifies the dilemmas generated by professionalization and bureaucratization and underscores the difficulties in balancing worker autonomy and personal risk taking with the protection of consumers and agencies.

Aronson and Neysmith (1996) differentiate the work of nursing aides and attendants in institutional settings from those in home care by noting that the home care worker's labor is less open to observation and regulation in the privacy of a care recipient's home. While this freedom has its positive dimensions, these researchers argue that workers in institutional settings have immediate supervisors and co-workers who have knowledge of the clients' needs and can help them in making important care decisions. In home care, where the worker is isolated in the home of a client, the caregiver feels moral responsibility for such decisions. In their study of home care workers and their supervisors, these researchers found that the supervisors had little time to support or monitor the frontline workers and that they also turned a blind eye to extra activities not within the workers' job descriptions. This lack of oversight allowed the home care aides to engage in some of the more interpersonal and off-duty tasks, but it also left them vulnerable to the whims of elderly clients and their families.

EMERGING HCBC TRENDS: ISSUES OF CARING

Within the arena of long-term care, two trends that emerged in the 1990s and that will help to shape the future of care are assisted living and "consumer direction" in home care. Both have the potential for encouraging as well as impeding the development of caring in the future.

Assisted Living

Policymakers, private developers, and consumers are focusing increased attention on the development of assisted-living facilities, environments that have some potential for encouraging the development of caring relationships. Some argue that *assisted living* is just a chic term for a setting that has been around for centuries. Homes for the aged, frequently associated with fraternal and religious organizations, proliferated in the nineteenth and early twentieth centuries to address the room-and-board needs of the poor and indigent infirm elderly. A modern version of homes for the aged is the relatively small board-and-care home. Such homes have become a refuge for the chronically mentally ill in response to the deinstitutionalization frenzy of the 1960s.

In the 1980s, the term *residential care facility* became fashionable for services that provided room, board, and some level of protective oversight. About half a million people in the United States live in licensed residential care facilities or board-and-care homes (Hawes, Wildfire, and Lux, 1993). Perhaps twice that number live in unlicensed facilities (Newcomer, Wilson, and Lee, 1997).

What appears to differentiate assisted living from the general concept of residential care and the somewhat pejorative label *board-and-care* is a matter of philosophy and emphasis on care as well as housing in assisted living (Kane, 1997). A recent survey of assisted-living regulations in fifty states indicates that four states use interchangeably the terms *assisted living* and *residential care* (Mollica and Snow, 1996). For the other states, key characteristics differentiating assisted living from other residential care models are:

—an explicit focus on autonomy, independence, and privacy (having a private room; the ability to lock doors; having a separate bath)

—an emphasis on apartment settings in which residents may choose to share living space
—the direct provision or arrangement of personal care and some nursing services—services that vary with level of disability and need

The assisted-living philosophy of autonomy and choice could have a positive or a negative impact on the degree of caring in a facility. On the one hand, an emphasis on a homelike environment free from the institutional trappings of a nursing home or other congregate setting could foster more human interaction and personal relationships between residents and staff; on the other hand, an emphasis on privacy and independence could isolate some residents and even lead to self-neglect or formal neglect through lack of attention and monitoring.

A national study of assisted living (Hawes, Rose, and Phillips, 1999) found that most facilities offer consumers a choice of privacy options: options might range from single rooms with private bath to one-bedroom, single-occupancy apartments. A majority of facilities were generally willing to serve residents who had moderate physical limitations, but fewer than half were willing to admit or retain residents who needed assistance with transferring from a bed or chair. Furthermore, fewer than half of the participating facilities would house residents with moderate to severe cognitive impairment, and only 28 percent would serve residents with behavioral symptoms such as wandering.

The study noted that residents of the facilities participating in the investigation had considerably more privacy and choice than did residents in most nursing homes and board-and-care homes the authors had studied previously. But it was also noted that there was much variability across facilities, and a substantial segment of the industry provided environments that did not appear consistent with the assisted-living philosophy. Furthermore, the large proportion of facilities with policies that excluded the cognitively impaired or severely physically disabled suggests that assisted living is not an environment where "aging in place" can occur for those who experience significant functional decline while they are residents.

Assisted-living facilities do have promise as environments that promote caring, but a number of impediments to the realization of this promise need serious attention. Currently, the assisted-living market is primarily for the well-to-do elderly; it is financially out of reach for moderate- or low-income individuals. The average monthly rate for facilities offering either high service or high privacy being $1,800 (Hawes, Rose, and

Phillips, 1999). Due, in part, to the limited sources and inadequacy of public financing, which could help to subsidize the room, board, and care costs for the financially strapped, those with moderate or low income have few options available.

There are also other impediments. For example, state policymakers and potential private providers have expressed concern about balancing consumer choice and privacy with health and safety and potential legal liability. The ambivalence toward regulating this market is a reflection of this ongoing struggle. On the one hand, there is the concern that without strong regulation and enforcement, consumers will be left to the whims of assisted-living providers. On the other hand, many advocates, as well as providers, fear that strict regulations (with a strong emphasis on structure and process) would undermine the privacy and autonomy philosophy of assisted living and its potential as a caring environment; that, they say, would simply recreate a nursing home industry.

There is also some question about the motivation of for-profit providers in the assisted-living industry. These providers are more likely to be developers and hotel managers than care providers, and when profit is the key catalyst the probability that a caring model will be encouraged is reduced. Furthermore, there has been concern that, as nursing homes look for new markets to deal with dwindling reimbursement and to circumvent government regulations, many skilled nursing facilities will simply lay down carpet, install doors with locks, and hang out the assisted-living shingle. Finally, despite the label, there is some question as to the amount of "assistance" that is actually provided in assisted-living facilities. According to the study by Hawes, Rose, and Phillips (1999), 65 percent of the participating facilities were categorized as "low service"; that is, they did not have an RN on staff or they did not provide nursing care (but did offer twenty-four-hour oversight, housekeeping, two meals, and some personal assistance). Another 5 percent were categorized as "minimal service" facilities in which personal assistance with ADLs was not offered. When coupled with the finding that many facilities do not accommodate people with significant cognitive or physical impairment, the concern that assisted living is "long on living" but "short on assistance" (and, perhaps, caring) seems warranted.

Consumer-Directed Care

The recent focus on consumer direction in HCBC may also have some potential for development of caring relationships, particularly among elderly consumers of care. Consumer direction has its roots in the independent-living movement of the 1970s. Working-age individuals with physical disabilities began to strongly oppose institutionalization; they advocated for home- and community-based options with consumers in control of hiring and firing their workers and in managing their services (Batavia, DeJong, and McKnew, 1991). Many of the younger disabled argued against the use of the term *care;* most were not sick; they needed personal "assistance" (rather than care) to remain independent in the community, including the workplace.

The distinction between care and assistance is important to understanding the impetus for consumer direction and the extent to which this concept is applicable to the disabled elderly population, including those with cognitive impairments. Many younger people with disabilities are interested in and willing to assume the complexity of responsibilities related to being an employer and managing their own services; they hire workers in the private marketplace and pay Social Security and Workmen's Compensation taxes. But the capacity and desire of older people—particularly today's elderly—to so intensively direct their own care is questionable, at least. If the consumer-direction concept is broadly defined as a continuum, ranging from a "direction lite" variety (i.e., simple involvement, of the consumer and the consumer's family in care planning and decision making) to the ultimate in consumer direction (providing cash benefits to beneficiaries and allowing them to purchase their own services), it is likely that many disabled elders would opt for "lite."

Much of the activity in the area of consumer direction at the state level has been through Medicaid HCBC waiver programs and state-funded personal-assistance services programs. California, for example, has a large independent provider program for elderly and younger disabled home care clients. Rather than receiving case-managed services through an agency, participants have the option of hiring and firing their own workers. As employers, they have the ability to direct their own care and to be more personally responsible for the quality of the care provided. The state maintains a registry of home care workers, but also allows clients to hire their own family members as caregivers.

The Medicaid program generally precludes direct cash payments to care recipients. However, through a demonstration and evaluation project, jointly funded by the U.S. Department of Health and Human Services and the Robert Wood Johnson Foundation, four states (New York, New Jersey, Arkansas, and Florida) are in various stages of securing Medicaid waivers to "cash out" the HCBC benefit. The states are currently designing their respective programs to include (1) establishment of cash payment rates; (2) development of marketing strategies to enroll a treatment and control group (those receiving case-managed agency services); (3) development of counseling programs to help recipients use the cash wisely and become good employers; and (4) creation of a quality monitoring system that preserves consumer autonomy while at the same time attempting to ensure safety and minimize fraud and abuse by clients and family members.

The results of this experiment will not be available for several years; however, a natural laboratory exists in Germany, where, since 1995, the state has been providing universal coverage for long-term care to disabled people of all ages. Recipients have the choice of several options, including a service package, a discounted cash benefit, or a combination of the two (Schneider, 1997). Statistics for the first year of operation indicated that 80 percent of care recipients with the lowest level of impairment and nearly two-thirds of the severely disabled (including a majority of the elderly beneficiaries) opted for cash benefits. Since the cash payments are considerably lower than the money-value of the service package, the overwhelming use of the cash option has helped keep the budget for this social-insurance program within prescribed limits. To date, there have been no evaluations of the effects of this program on quality of care, but the Germans do not appear to be as obsessed as Americans with the potential for fraud and abuse or undue harm to beneficiaries.

Interest in promoting a caring paradigm was not part of the official rhetoric that surrounded the enactment of this German program. Rather, the flexibility in benefits that it offered was designed to save costs as well as to provide more choice to people with long-term care needs and their family caregivers. Yet the opportunity to choose one's own professional caregivers and to direct one's own care might help to foster more personal interaction and caring relationships between care recipients and workers who are not constrained by a bureaucratic agency. At the same time, however, the potential for enhanced caring must be weighed against the potential for abuse by caregivers or worker abuse perpetrated by care recipients.

As consumer direction becomes more familiar to policymakers as well as providers and various subpopulations, it will be interesting to see the extent to which this model becomes a major option in public policy. Historically, U.S. policymakers have been comfortable with a cash-benefit approach for certain groups (e.g., the working disabled, and veterans). They have been less sanguine about direct payments to potentially "undeserving" individuals such as SSI beneficiaries, as is reflected in Congressional actions to reduce or eliminate benefits for certain groups of disabled children and substance abusers. Concerns about the misuse of dollars as well as potential liability in the face of unforeseen mishaps have impeded the growth of this trend in the United States. At the same time, younger people with disabilities have begun to join forces with advocates for older persons to fight for more choice and autonomy in HCBC.

Consumer direction is not an option for all people with long-term care needs, but it may prove to be an effective and efficient way to allocate precious resources to an important subset of the population. Depending on the perspective from which it is viewed, consumer-directed programs can be seen as a relatively safe and inexpensive way to satisfy consumer needs and allow payment to relatives and friends for important service delivery, or as a vehicle for depressing wages, exploiting workers, and jeopardizing the health and well-being of vulnerable consumers (Feldman, 1997).

The issue of caring has not been an explicit part of the debate so far. But embedded in the concerns about the safety and quality of care for consumers and the potential abuse and exploitation of the workers is the worry that caring is less likely to occur in the consumer-directed model. Caring and consumer direction are not mutually exclusive; in fact, the potential for caring could be enhanced in a situation where the disabled person was given choice of caregiver and where there was no agency or bureaucracy discouraging the relational aspects of care. The "worker as stranger" could become the "worker as fictive kin" (Karner, 1998), with the increased possibility of developing and nurturing the intimacy that is required to provide quality HCBC.

Elderly consumers are probably more likely to prefer a caring approach and to operationalize consumer direction within this paradigm. Younger people with disabilities who view themselves as employers and their personal care attendants as strictly employees (Eustis and Fischer, 1991) may not be interested in the caring aspect. In fact, they may even view such an approach as antithetical to the independent-living philosophy. If the pure employment model is to be successful, both care recipient and caregiver must reject the relational caring paradigm.

TOWARD A CARING PARADIGM

As America ages and the longevity revolution among the younger disabled continues, we are likely to see the demand for more long-term care

HCBC options in the future, as well as a continuing need for subacute care in the home. Many will want to live as independently as possible for as long as possible in their own homes, relying on a varying combination of informal and formal care, assistive technology, and community-based supports such as adult day care. Others will choose a congregate setting, where the promise of a good roof over one's head, a community of peers based on age or other common characteristics, and service availability converge to provide comfort and safety. As this chapter has emphasized, however, the need for care and support changes continually, and a dynamic, flexible system must be available and affordable to meet the needs of very diverse populations over time. And for some, HCBC may not be the appropriate option—either for the care recipient or the family.

Regardless of the care setting and modality, it is clear that the caring dimension has, to a greater or lesser extent, been lost in the evolution of HCBC from a purely private family or neighborhood activity to a formal enterprise with standards, regulations, and profits. And for some families, caring may never have been part of the family dynamic. Consequently, "policymakers ought to worry about . . . the displacement of caring relationships and social connections by narrow, task-oriented bodily maintenance; the displacement of empathy and affection by cool professionalism and calculated fiscal prudence; and the displacement of an ethic of responsibility for one's neighbors by an ethic of working-to-rule" (Stone, 1999: 67).

As the HCBC policy debate continues into the next century, we must make sure that it does not just focus on how to finance care. The issues of designing a caring, humane delivery system must be a priority as well. In examining how policy might make it more likely that people will want to undertake caring for others, we must address the training requirements of both the professional and paraprofessional workers in long-term care. The caring dimension must be introduced and encouraged through formal education and on-the-job training. The relational aspects of care must be rewarded, both monetarily and spiritually, so that workers continue to be motivated to engage in the most important noninstrumental tasks of caring.

This caring system, however, must start with the person needing care and her or his family. In that caring dyad, both the care recipient and the caregiver must understand that the dynamics of care provision tend to mirror the dynamics of their personal relationship. They must learn to embrace a model of accommodation and reciprocity and, also, to recognize when the informal care alternative is no longer a viable and appropriate option.

REFERENCES

Abel, E. K. (1991). *Who Cares for the Elderly? Public Policy and the Experiences of Adult Daughters.* Philadelphia, PA: Temple University Press.

Aronson, J., and Neysmith, S. M. (1996). "You're not just in there to do the work": Depersonalizing policies and the exploitation of home care workers' labor. *Gender and Society* 10(1): 59–77.

Arras, J. D., and Dubler, N. N. (1995). Introduction: Ethical and social implications of high-tech home care. In J. D. Arras, ed., *Bringing the Hospital Home: Ethical and Social Implications of High-Tech Home Care,* pp. 1–31. Baltimore: Johns Hopkins University Press.

Aulisio, M. P., May, T., and Aulisio, M. S. (1998). Vulnerabilities of clients and caregivers in the home care setting. *Generations* 22(3): 58–63.

Baines, C. T., Evans, P. M., and Neysmith, S. M. (1991). Caring: Its impact on the lives of women. In C. Baines, P. M. Evans, and S. M. Neysmith, eds., *Women's Caring,* pp. 11–35. Toronto: McClelland & Stewart. Cited by MacRae, 1998.

Batavia, A. I., DeJong, G., and McKnew, L. B. (1991). Toward a national personal assistance program: The independent living model of long term care for persons with disabilities. *Journal of Health Politics, Policy, and Law* 16(3): 523–45.

Bayer, R. (1986). Ethical challenges in the movement for home health care. *Generations* 10(4): 44–47.

Binstock, R. H., and Cluff, L. E. (2000). Issues and challenges in home care. In R. H. Binstock and L. W. Cluff, eds., *Home Care Advances: Essential Research and Policy Issues,* pp. 3–34. New York: Springer Publishing.

Branch, L. G., Coulam, R. F., and Zimmerman, Y. A. (1995). The PACE evaluation: Initial findings. *Gerontologist* 35: 349–59.

Brody, E. M. (1985). Parent care as a normative family stress. *Gerontologist* 25: 19–29.

Brown, M. A., and Stetz, K. (1999). The labor of caregiving: A theoretical model of caregiving during potentially fatal illness. *Qualitative Health Research* 9(2): 182–97.

Burwell, B. (1999). *Medicaid Long Term Care Expenditures in FY 1998.* Memorandum, April 14. Cambridge, MA: MedStat Group.

Clement, G. (1996). *Care, Autonomy, and Justice: Feminism and the Ethic of Care.* Boulder, CO: Westview Press.

Collopy, B., Dubler, N., and Zuckerman, C. (1990). The ethics of home care: Autonomy and accommodation. *Hastings Center Report* 20(2): 1–16.

Eustis, N. N., and Fischer, L. R. (1991). Relationships between home care clients and their workers: Implications for quality of care. *Gerontologist* 31(4): 447–56.

Feldman, P. H. (1997). Labor market issues in home care. In D. M. Fox and C. Raphael, eds., *Home-Based Care for a New Century,* pp. 15–183. Malden, MA: Blackwell.

Glasser, R., and Brecker, J. (1997). We are the roots: The culture of home health aides. *New England Journal of Public Policy* 13(1): 113–34.

Hawes, C., Rose, M., and Phillips, C. D. (1999). *A National Study of Assisted Living for the Frail Elderly: Results of a National Survey of Facilities.* Beachwood, OH: Menorah Park Center for the Aging.

Hawes, C., Wildfire, J. B., and Lux, L. J. (1993). *Regulation of Board and Care Homes: Results of a Survey in the 50 States and the District of Columbia: National Summary.* Washington, DC: American Association of Retired Persons.

Kane, R. A. (1997). Boundaries of home care: Can a home-care approach transform LTC institutions? In D. M. Fox and C. Raphael, eds., *Home-Based Care for a New Century,* pp. 23–46. Malden, MA: Blackwell.

Kane, R. A., Kane, R. L., and Ladd, R. C. (1998). *The Heart of Long-Term Care.* New York: Oxford University Press.

Karner, T. X. (1998). Professional caring: Home care worker as fictive kin. *Journal of Aging Studies* 12(1): 69–82.

Komisar, H. L., Lambrew, J. M., and Feder, J. (1996). *Long-Term Care for the Elderly.* New York: Commonwealth Fund.

Kuhn, D. R. (1998). Is homecare always the best care? *Generations* 22(3): 99–101.

Lillesto, B. (1997). Violation in caring for the physically disabled. *Western Journal of Nursing Research* 19(3): 282–96.

MacRae, H. (1998). Managing feelings: Caregiving as emotion work. *Research on Aging* 20(1): 137–60.

Mollica, R. L. (1998). *State Assisted Living Policy: 1998.* Washington, DC: Office of the Assistant Secretary for Planning and Evaluation, U.S. Department of Health and Human Services.

Mollica, R. L., and Snow, K. I. (1996). *State Assisted Living Policy: 1996.* Report prepared under contract DHHS-100-94-0044 for the U.S. Department of Health and Human Services, Washington, DC.

Moore, P. C., and McCollough, R. H. (2000). Hospice: End-of-life care. In R. H. Binstock and L. E. Cluff, eds., *Home Care Advances: Essential Research and Policy Issues,* pp. 101–16. New York: Springer Publishing.

National Adult Day Services Association: NADSA (1999). *Adult Day Services Fact Sheet.* http://www.ncoa.org/nadsa/ADS_factsheet.htm (with information also provided to the author orally by Mary Brugger Murphy at NADSA, May 13, 1999).

Newcomer, R. J., and Stone, R. I. (1985). Board and care housing: Expansion and improvement needed. *Generations* 10(3): 38–39.

Newcomer, R. J., Wilson, K. B., and Lee, P. (1997). Residential care for the frail elderly: State innovations in placement, financing, and governance. In R. J. Newcomer, A. M. Wilkinson, and M. P. Lawton, eds., *Annual Review of Gerontology and Geriatrics,* vol. 16, pp. 162–82. New York: Springer Publishing.

Noddings, N. (1984). *Caring: A Feminine Approach to Ethics and Moral Education.* Berkeley: University of California Press.

Noddings, N. (1995). Moral obligations or moral support for high-tech home care? In J. D. Arras, ed., *Bringing the Hospital Home: Ethical and Social Implications of High-Tech Home Care,* pp. 149–65. Baltimore: Johns Hopkins University Press.

Quinn, M. J., and Tomita, S. K. (1997). *Elder Abuse and Neglect: Causes, Diagnosis, and Intervention Strategies.* New York: Springer Publishing.

Rubinstein, R. L. (1990). Culture and disorder in the home care experience: The home as sickroom. In J. F. Gubrium and A. Sankar, eds., *The Home Care Experience: Ethnography and Policy,* pp. 37–57. Newbury Park, CA: Sage.

Schneider, U. (1997). *Germany's New Long-Term Care Policy: Profile and Assessment of the Social Dependency Insurance.* Policy paper #5 of the American Institute for Contemporary German Studies. Washington, DC: Johns Hopkins University.

Sixsmith, A. J. (1990). The meaning and experience of "home" in later life. In B. Bytheway and J. Johnson, eds., *Welfare and the Ageing Experience: A Multidisciplinary Analysis.* Aldershot, UK: Avebury. Cited in Twigg, 1997.

Stone, D. (1999). Care and trembling. *The American Prospect* 43 (March–April): 61–67.

Stone, R. I. (2000). *Long-Term Care for the Disabled Elderly: Current Policy. Emerging Trends, and Implications for the 21st Century.* New York: Milbank Memorial Fund (also available at www.milbank.org/stoneindex.html).

Tronto, J. C. (1998). An ethic of care. *Generations* 22(3): 15–20.

Twigg, J. (1997). Deconstructing the "social bath": Help with bathing at home for older and disabled people. *Journal of Social Policy* 26(2): 211–32.

9

Caring and Community-Based Voluntary Organizations

LINDA K. GEORGE, PH.D.

For most of my childhood, I lived in a small rural farming community. The "downtown" consisted of a hardware, feed, and seed store; a general store; a branch bank; a barbershop; a grange hall; two churches; and a volunteer fire department. Max lived at the firehouse. There was something wrong with Max; he wasn't "right." I was told that he had lived with his mother until she died and then the guys at the fire department fixed him up with a room and shower there. All the children were told to stay away from Max, but we certainly watched him. He collected piles of rocks; he had no favorite types of rocks—any rocks would do. He didn't talk much to others, but he had conversations with himself that didn't make sense to us. Most of the time, Max just hung around the firehouse or one of the stores.

Everyone took care of Max. Women of the community showed up several times a day with a small pot of homemade soup, freshly baked bread, tomatoes from the garden, or whatever. Farmers often picked him up and took him home for the day, where he would look for rocks while the hay was baled, the cows milked, and the stables cleaned. At night, there were usually at least a couple men at the firehouse; Max was there, though he paid little attention to the conversation. When one of the churches had a social or a potluck dinner, someone went and got Max, making sure he had on a clean flannel shirt and bib overalls. Max made out like a bandit at Christmas, receiving stacks of shirts, underwear, overalls, socks, gloves, and hats. When I left for college, Max was still there, seeming the same as always. Max was just, well, Max.

So, I grew up in a pastoral paradise à la Norman Rockwell, right?

Hardly. I was miserable in that little town where all 150-plus adults knew everything I did and had the right to tell me what and what not to do. I was known for asking stupid questions and keeping my head "buried in a book." It goes without saying that I had no common sense. My poor chances of ever marrying if I didn't "change my ways" were probably not the main issue on people's minds, but it seemed like that to me. I couldn't wait to leave that town and I have not been back since the day I left for college. Thankfully, my family moved to another community shortly after I left.

Max and I experienced the best and worst of a small, close-knit community. Max had the best—if you were one of "ours," no matter if you were dependent and incompetent, you were taken care of and treated like family. There was never any talk of sending Max away. There was never any talk of him being a burden or an embarrassment. I experienced the worst of such a community, suffering from its narrowness and self-righteousness and feeling like a misfit. I could tell Hillary Clinton a few things about what can happen when a village raises a child.

This chapter is about communities and the potential for community organizations to make significant contributions to human caring. Many of the chapters in this volume make the point that there is too little caring in our society—a situation that is a disservice to both those who need care and to the humanity of those who fail to provide it. In general, I agree with this assessment of our society. Memories of my childhood, however, lead me to ask a more complex question than simply how we can foster caring for those who suffer. I also want to determine whether we can foster caring at the community or voluntary-organization level that precludes the types of costs that are often exacted on members of such communities and organizations. In short, can community organizations provide care that matches the needs of the recipient, even when those needs are at odds with the care provider's view of what is good and true?

THE MEANING OF COMMUNITY

A well-known U.S. dictionary (*Webster's New Universal,* 1979) offers six definitions of community; all of them are based on geographic criteria (e.g., living in the same environment, living in the same society, being subjected to the same laws). Initially, sociologists, too, viewed communities as geographic units; indeed, social ecology was a primary perspective of early sociological studies in the United States (Tomasi, 1998). More recently, however, social scientists (e.g., McMillan and Chavis, 1986; Sarason, 1976) have backed away from a geography-based definition and focused on community as a collective of individuals who share common interests, goals, and, to at least some degree, identity. Such collectives may or may not be geographically based. The evolution of the term *community* occurred for several reasons. In part, a definition that required geographical boundaries was probably always overly restrictive. In addition, however, social change altered the frequency and importance of communities that transcend geographic boundaries. With modern means of communication, it is possible to be part of communities that have no geographic base. Most academicians, for example, probably view their scholarly community as extending far beyond the geographic confines of their own colleges and universities.

For our purposes, I will rely on the definition of community that refers to a collective of individuals who share common interests, goals, and a sense of shared identity. Communities meeting this definition may or may not be geographically based. It is likely that a large proportion of Americans do not "live" in communities—that is, their sense of community does not rest on where they reside. Some Americans may feel they are not part of any community. Most Americans, however, undoubtedly are members of communities that are not geographically based. One can belong to a multiplicity of communities (whether or not they are geographically based), which raises issues of varying levels of commitment across them.

Although communities need not be geographically based, it is doubtful that they can exist in the absence of some kind of organizational structure. Part of my personal identity may be based on my devotion to reading classical literature, but I cannot secure a sense of community or social identity from that activity without an organized group of other people with similar interests. Voluntary organizations provide an ideal setting for both geographically based and, especially, communities that are not geographically based. Indeed, the voluntary organization, which all of us take for granted, is a clever invention. Ideally, such an organization provides the structure needed to sustain a sense of community and accomplish shared goals. At the same time, because it is voluntary, no one is forced to participate or to suffer involuntarily from the organization's rules and expectations. This is quite different from the experience of growing up in a community in which one shares neither a sense of identity nor values.

The United States has long been known for its plethora of voluntary organizations. This country was founded, in part, on the desire of religious communities to pursue their faith and their mores without external interference. In the late 1700s, de Tocqueville was stunned by the number of voluntary organizations in this new country and intrigued by the functions they served for both individuals and the broader society (de Tocqueville [1835] 1956; see also chapter 11). Voluntary organizations remain a major part of our society, and many Americans belong, with varying levels of commitment, to one or more organizations (see e.g., Curtis, Grabb, and Baer, 1992).

THE UNIQUE CHARACTERISTICS OF VOLUNTARY ORGANIZATIONS

There is a vast literature on voluntary organizations and it is unnecessary to review it here. But in this section I will highlight the structural facets and tendencies of voluntary organizations that are most likely to affect their ability to be significant sources of caring.

The fact that voluntary organizations are voluntary is both their greatest strength and their primary weakness. The voluntary aspect benefits both the members and the organization itself: the individual can leave the organization at will and without penalty (a characteristic that makes voluntary organizations less coercive than most other social structures); and the voluntarism is an advantage for the organization because members, presumably, have some level of commitment to it or they would not remain members. Another strength of voluntary organizations is that they can be established quickly, to meet sudden or suddenly recognized needs (another characteristic not typical of most social structures). Voluntary organizations can set their own priorities, policies, and activities, with few restrictions. And they can change course quickly because they are accountable only to their members. In short, voluntary organizations have a higher level of flexibility than is characteristic of most other forms of organizations and social structures.

But voluntary organizations have structural disadvantages as well. Substantial time, energy, and commitment are required to establish a voluntary organization, and these demands typically are shared by very few individuals, at least initially. As a result, many voluntary organizations never really get off the ground, faltering before they become established and have a critical mass of members. Even among established voluntary organizations there is considerable instability (Thompson, 1967; Zucker, 1988). Because of the high rate of organizational demise, members that remain active usually must devote a large part of their effort to recruiting new members. A final and major limitation of voluntary organizations is their lack of authority over the membership. Voluntary organizations can reward exemplary members (although the rewards are usually more symbolic than tangible), but they can do little to punish those that err beyond verbal censure and expulsion. Apathy and a low level of commitment are common problems in voluntary organizations and there is little that organizations can do to obviate them beyond making persuasive appeals (Murnigham, Kim, and Metzer, 1993; Omoto and Snyder, 1995).

It also is important to note that voluntary organizations have a life course—that they change over time. To some degree, this happens in predictable ways. Social scientists use the term *institutionalization* to refer to the processes by which social structures change (e.g., DiMaggio and Powell, 1983; Powell, 1985). There are strong incentives for these processes to occur since they are strongly associated with organizational survival. The primary purpose of institutionalization is to create a stable, viable organization that is equipped to survive. The primary methods by which institutionalization accomplishes this purpose are bureaucratization, routinization, and implementation of procedures to insure survival, and perhaps growth. Thus, over time, organizational policies and procedures become standardized and routinized. Leadership becomes organized along lines of official rights and responsibilities. Protecting the organization, as opposed to pursuing its goals, becomes a core activity. Bureaucratization and routinization typically take the forms of formal bylaws, the implemention of a leadership structure, and the handling of meetings in a formal style, with an explicit agenda. A number of methods can be used to sustain organizational survival (see, e.g., Scott, 1995; Zucker, 1988). Recruitment of new members is usually a key strategy. Other methods can include a formal dues structure, accumulation of financial reserves, and explicit fund-raising efforts. As an organization grows, additional forms of institutionalization may include incorporation as a nonprofit organization, the hiring of paid staff, appointing or electing a board of directors, and securing professional help such as accounting or legal services.

Institutionalization poses a paradox for voluntary organizations. On the one hand, it is often a prerequisite for survival and for routinizing the means of survival. On the other hand, institutionalization decreases flexibility, which is one of voluntary organizations' greatest strengths and most distinctive characteristics. Moreover, institutionalization can become an end rather than a means—the end of organizational efforts rather than the means to accomplish the organization's purpose. In other forms of organizations there are pressures to keep institutionalization within reasonable bounds. For example, if businesses are to survive, they must achieve an appropriate balance between institutionalization and serving their clients. This is not the case for voluntary organizations. Although, in all likelihood, voluntary organizations that accomplish nothing other than institutionalization are unlikely to survive over the long term, it can take a very long time for this to occur. Some can survive indefinitely, however, reflecting a disproportionate commitment to survival and little purpose beyond that.

VOLUNTARY ORGANIZATIONS AND CARING

The Meaning of Caring

Before evaluating the potential role that voluntary organizations can play in caring, I will briefly recap what Daniel Callahan says about caring in chapter 1: (a) caring is focused on the needs of the recipient; (b) caring is offered regardless of the probability that the recipient will recover what he or she has lost; (c) caring is aimed at psychological and spiritual needs, as well as purely physical ones; (d) caring addresses both the general and specific needs of recipients; (e) caring is relational; (f) caring focuses primarily upon alleviating suffering. In this chapter, these dimensions define what I mean by caring.

In caring, meeting the above criteria is not an easy task. Indeed, it is not clear that many individuals have the sensitivity, objectivity, and endurance to provide this kind of caring. I am struck by the similarity between caring, as defined by Callahan, and nondirective, supportive therapy as it is defined by mental health professionals. It is worth noting that psychotherapists require lengthy training and experience to practice supportive therapy. In my view, many components of Callahan's definition of caring are not within the control of voluntary organizations. In practical terms, these organizations cannot ensure that the interactions between care providers and recipients are characterized by a focus on the patients' needs, meet psychological and spiritual as well as physical needs, and so forth. The components of Callahan's definition do, however, appear to have two possible links with voluntary organizations: the training of individuals to provide high-quality caring; and in fostering caring relationships. Both of these I address below.

The Match and Mismatch of Voluntary Organizations and Caring

The structural characteristics of voluntary organizations highlight the potential and problems of relying upon them for caring, although, in number, if not in substantive effects, the strengths outweigh the weaknesses.

One advantage of voluntary organizations is their flexibility. Unlike formal health and social service agencies, voluntary organizations *need* not be constrained by formal eligibility criteria, limits on the range and amount of services provided, rigid fee schedules, and issues of "turf." Many voluntary organizations do, it is true, develop formal policies concerning these matters, but even then they have the flexibility to change the policies at will and to grant exemptions from the policies. In the formal service network, fragmentation of services is characteristic, whereas voluntary organizations do not have to propagate fragmentation: they are free to develop a service program that best suits the needs of caring recipients and help recipients to access other services more efficiently and comfortably.

Caring services provided by voluntary organizations are also likely to have an individual element that benefits both care provider and recipient. Care providers often experience a sense of meaning and self-worth from helping to alleviate the suffering of others (see, e.g., Piliavin and Charng, 1990; Wilson and Janowski, 1995). In addition, they often view their contributions as an investment in their own futures. They may not and cannot expect a specific reward in return, but they often feel that by providing caring they increase the likelihood that caring will be there for them when it is needed. Care recipients often value the caring that they receive from volunteers because it often seems more genuine than that provided by formal agencies: volunteer providers are there because they want to be, not because it is their job. Caring provided by volunteers, compared with that provided by formal agencies, also is less likely to make recipients feel dependent or like charity cases, and it may seem less like a burdensome obligation than that provided by friends and family. Moreover, recipients know that they can reject the efforts of volunteer care providers in ways less awkward than with either formal providers or friends and family.

The biggest potential problem with voluntary organizations as caring providers is their inherent risk of instability. This instability can occur at multiple levels. At the organizational level, organizations can disband or change their priorities, perhaps ending successful caring programs; this may leave other organizations struggling to fill the gap and care recipients with a sense of rejection. Some organizations pursue multiple activities and are unwilling to provide the level of commitment to caring that is required for a successful program. Then, when care recipients (whether individuals or organizations) decline their offers to provide care, the voluntary organization is confused or resentful. Instability at the level of individual members is also a common problem for voluntary organizations. The literature on voluntary organizations and volunteerism consistently finds that volunteer drop-out and poor performance (e.g., not showing up, behaving in inappropriate ways) are persistent problems (Murnigham, Kim, and Metzer, 1993; Omoto and Snyder, 1995).

Nuts-and-Bolts Issues

I suspect that voluntary organizations can play a significant caring role only under specific conditions. First, caring must be a major mission and commitment of the organization. Caring is fragile, and I doubt it can survive within an organization if it has to vie for its existence with other projects, intense membership drives, and aggressive fund-raising. Caring requires putting other things aside and focusing on feelings, listening, relinquishing judgment and prejudice, and making a commitment of time and energy to a relationship. That relationship may be a relatively short one, but it is intense, and if it is to succeed the care provider must be dependable. Unless a voluntary organization, as a unit, and its members, as individuals, are willing to make caring a high priority, caring relationships cannot be established and sustained.

Many voluntary organizations take on time-limited service projects, such as delivering holiday presents to the needy or making occasional visits to nursing homes (often en masse, for a celebration of some kind). These services undoubtedly benefit the recipients, but they do not constitute caring as Callahan has so wisely defined it. Caring relationships are unlikely to develop via such brief interaction. Moreover, the services are chosen by the organization; they may or may not meet some general needs of the recipients, but it is *certain* that they do not serve recipients' specific, personal needs. Caring is different from other services provided by voluntary organizations; it requires special kinds of relationships between care providers and recipients.

One area where voluntary organizations could enhance caring is in teaching volunteers to provide high-quality caring. Callahan's criteria for caring are specific and require attitudes and behaviors that are different from most other forms of social interaction. Indeed, I doubt that most interactions among family members meet his criteria for caring. But individuals can learn what caring is and how best to establish and sustain caring relationships. Developing appropriate training programs for care providers would be an important contribution to society and one that voluntary organizations are in an ideal position to make.

Such training programs need to be substantially different from traditional forms of volunteer training. I have attended several such training programs and I find that most focus much more on issues such as the importance of showing up on time, paperwork, politeness, and potential legal liability than on how the trainees can best help to alleviate suffering while maintaining the individual's autonomy and dignity. Effective training programs would also help trainees in deciding whether they are willing and able to make the kind of commitment that caring relationships require.

CARING ORGANIZATIONS: SOME ILLUSTRATIONS

Very few organizations make a substantial commitment to caring—at least, not in the terms of the definition detailed above. Moreover, there is no research that has evaluated the success of specific organizations or types of organizations in providing such caring. In this section, I briefly describe four types of organizations that *appear* to have had success in caring for others, although the research base does not specifically address caring. This is not to say that these types of organizations always provide caring or succeed in their attempts to do so, but they do view caring as a central part of their mission, and they do apparently often succeed in providing it.

Religious Organizations

Most religious groups view caring for group members as a sacred responsibility (Luks and Payne, 1992; Wilson and Janowski, 1995). Alleviating suffering, helping those less fortunate, providing comfort and solace, and finding meaning in suffering are responsibilities that most churches take very seriously (here and throughout, I use the terms *church* and *churches* generically, to include all types of religious organizations). Caring for each other in a church is the responsibility of everyone—not only church leadership, but also the general membership, although there may be groups designated with overall responsibility for some aspects of care.

In addition to their moral commitment to caring, churches are ideal organizations for the effective provision of care. Churches are communities—communities of faith. Church members typically know one another, often for long periods of time. They have worshiped together, participated in church-sponsored activities, and shared each other's celebrations and griefs, often with formal rites of passage. Caring relationships are often a structural element of religious organizations; members take it for granted that a good congregation provides care for its members. They expect to provide care to other members and they expect to receive care when they are in need. There is no charity in this. Caring is not a formal service; it is part of the very fabric of the religious community.

Church members obviously differ in the extent to which they participate in caring relationships with other members. But the religious community takes caring seriously and typically backs up its beliefs with appropriate action. As in other forms of integrated communities, the mission is separate from the desires of individual church members. This is not the kind of supportive care offered by families, who may die off, become estranged, or simply become exhausted by the physical demands of care. Religious caring is the responsibility of the religious community, and if members die, leave, or are unable to respond, other members are there to fill community duties.

Caring provided by religious groups has another benefit as well: church members not only share a history of activities, but also a worldview (see, e.g., Allport, 1950). There is history of discussing the most profound and challenging parts of life—how to live with grief and disappointment, the need to be thankful for one's blessings, how to forgive and be forgiven, how to live a good life, how to accept oneself, how to find the courage to make or accept change. Given this history of both behavior and shared concerns, caring relationships typically develop smoothly and naturally, and the shared identity of true communities can be taken for granted, rather than needing to be established.

I am not claiming that all churches succeed at nurturing caring relationships or that all church members receive appropriate caring from their congregations. Compared with most organizations, however, churches are in an ideal position to undertake caring for their members—and in a way that is likely to be comfortable and comforting to both care providers and care receivers.

One-on-One Programs

Some organizations sponsor one-on-one programs in which group members develop close relationships with a person in need. Big Brothers and Big Sisters are examples of this kind of program. But one-on-one programs are common in many voluntary organizations (e.g., becoming companions to nursing home patients or homebound individuals, intensive tutoring programs, mentoring programs). One-on-one programs have great potential for engendering caring relationships. Beyond the obvious advantage of a program based on sustained dyadic relationships, group members who commit to a one-on-one relationship understand what is involved and are willing to engage in a level of intimacy different from that of "service projects."

One-on-one programs have a solid history of success, as measured by the satisfaction levels of participants (on both sides), behavior change, and the tangible accomplishments of the care recipient, and the fact that these relationships often continue long after the formal obligations are complete (see, e.g., Pancoast, Parker, and Froland, 1983; Skirboll and Pavelsky, 1984; for an exception, however, see Cohen, Hyland, and Devlin, 1999). I have some concerns, however, about the status discrepancies in many one-to-one programs between volunteers and the individuals with whom they develop relationships. Unless these relationships are handled carefully, the agenda pursued will be that of the volunteer rather than that of the individual who is to receive support. Apparently this has not been a problem in programs such as Big Brothers and Big Sisters, where status differences—and perhaps the volunteer's right to set the agenda for shared activities, frequency of contact, and so on—are an accepted part of the program. I am unaware, however, of one-on-one programs that have focused sensitively on the issues faced by chronically or terminally ill persons or those who experience other forms of suffering. In those situations, for one-on-one relationships to be helpful, I believe the focus needs to be on the care recipient's concerns and personal agenda.

Support Groups

Over the last twenty-five years, support groups have become a significant component of the voluntary-organization sector. There are support groups focused on nearly every illness and problem imaginable. Support groups take a variety of forms. Some are purely "grass roots"; others are established and directed by other organizations, often health or social service agencies. Some support groups focus exclusively on sharing concerns and receiving support; others make a substantial commitment to educational efforts (e.g., getting information from experts on the disease or problem and finding strategies to handle it). The common element of support groups is that they are composed of persons who all face or have faced a specific type of problem or issue: it is widely believed that support received from others who share or have shared one's situation is qualitatively different from the support provided by those who have not experienced that problem.

Research gives good marks to support groups (e.g., Greene and Monahan, 1989; Levy, Derby, and Martinkowski, 1993; Toseland, Rossiter, and Labrecque, 1989). It is clear that support-group members typically are highly satisfied with their experience and find comfort and support from their participation. Evidence regarding the educational benefits of support groups is less clear, but is also less relevant from the perspective of caring.

I have two concerns about support groups. First, the research indicates that large numbers of individuals attend support groups once or twice and do not return (Lieberman, Borman, and Associates, 1979; Silverman, 1980). These individuals have not been included in the evaluation studies, so the evidence of the benefits of support-group participation is limited to those members who choose to remain active participants. Presumably, a large proportion of the individuals who never become members of support groups did not find their needs met by this type of organization. Second, and based on my professional opinion rather than research, I have concerns about support groups' exclusive focus on a single aspect of members' lives. No label or condition (e.g., cancer patient; cancer survivor; compulsive eater; gambler) captures the rich complexity of a human life. I am confident that a form of caring occurs in support groups; I am less confident that the caring meets all the criteria used in this chapter.

Small Homogeneous Communities

There is not, so far as I know, a magic number of individuals that a collectivity must reach in order to qualify as a community. And my sense is that, for purposes of caring, smaller communities are better than larger ones. I think caring communities are not very common. Certainly the small rural community where I was raised did not qualify as one: it served people well so long as they fit expectations, but had no tolerance for questions or for failure to conform, and no recognition of suffering beyond physical pain and material need. Caring communities do exist, however—and since most seem to reflect the values of their members rather than explicit intentions to develop caring communities, I find them commendable and intriguing.

Evidence for caring communities comes from a variety of ethnographic studies, and it is doubtful that they could be revealed by any other methodology. Many of these studies are of older people living in shared environments such as a retirement community (e.g., Hochschild, 1973; Matthews, 1979; Rubinstein, 1986). But there are many others as well, such as Stack's poignant description of a small, poor, African American community in the deep South (Stack, 1974). The communities described in these studies are invariably small and socially homogeneous, though not all of them (e.g., retirement communities) were characterized by long-term relationships among group members.

Not all small communities are caring communities. This is documented especially well by Kanter in her study of communes that endure and those that fail (Kanter, 1972). The three factors she identified as increasing the probability of survival were (1) a shared ideology, (2) shared social characteristics, and (3) a balance of intimacy and respect among commune members. It seems to me that these factors also increase the likelihood of caring relationships.

Encouraging the development of caring communities is a dubious pursuit. It is not clear that one can mandate or even significantly increase the probability that community members will form the social ties required for a caring community. Moreover, there are undoubtedly a variety of circumstances that preclude development of a sense of community (e.g., too little shared ideology or social characteristics, or an impaired population that lacks the health and vitality to forge a sense of community). In addition, the mechanisms, such as social homogeneity, that seem to facilitate caring communities are contrary to current political standards (e.g., it is hard, these days, to build a retirement community that is explicitly homogeneous in terms of race, education, and religion). Although there is not much that can be done to provide incentives for the development of caring communities, we can certainly support such communities when they develop naturally, and celebrate the rewards that such communities provide to their members.

THE INTERFACE BETWEEN THE VOLUNTARY SECTOR AND FORMAL AGENCIES

Voluntary organizations occupy a unique niche in the range of social structures with the potential to provide caring. But their caring activities should be compatible with those provided by other kinds of organizations; at least, they should not be in competition with or undermine them. One implication of this is the need for an effective interface between voluntary organizations and formal service organizations.

I am not aware of any research documenting the extent to which voluntary organizations typically have formal or informal relationships with community service agencies or the conditions under which such relationships are more or less effective. There seem to be a number of issues, however, that have the potential to affect the quality and success of the relationships between voluntary organizations and community agencies.

Most important, voluntary organizations need to be aware of the ways in which their activities might duplicate community agencies' mandates and programs; they need to communicate with the agencies their recognition of such issues and focus their activities appropriately. Community agencies are highly sensitive to issues of turf and often do not welcome a service that appears to compete with or duplicate what they do. In the current economic and political environment, community agencies often are struggling for their very existence. Part of justifying their existence is the ability to demonstrate that they are providing critical services that are not otherwise available. Thus, if a voluntary organization establishes programs that duplicate or even appear to duplicate an agency's efforts, the organization may well be viewed as a threat or a competitor. Under these conditions, an effective relationship between the community agency and the voluntary organization is unlikely, if not impossible. But if voluntary organizations do what they are best equipped and ideally positioned to do, there should be minimal overlap with the programs provided by community agencies. Below, I list six ways in which voluntary organizations can usefully provide important services. The final three are interrelated and speak directly to caring, as distinct from provision of specific services.

1. Voluntary organizations can play an important role in channeling or referring appropriate individuals to community service programs (see, e.g., Halpert, 1988). Such outreach benefits both the agencies and the individuals who are not receiving, or who are not even aware of, available services. It is important, however, that members of voluntary organizations always discuss the matter with the individuals concerned before referring them to the community agency—not merely out of politeness but also to honor the autonomy and authority of the individual being "helped."

2. There are always gaps between the needs of potential care recipients and the range of community services available. These gaps are the ideal sites for voluntary organizations to develop programs. Such programs complement rather than duplicate agency services.

3. Voluntary organizations can target individuals who are "ineligible" for services from community agencies. Most agencies are able to serve

only those individuals who meet multiple eligibility criteria, ranging from level of disability to income. Typically, there are many more individuals who would benefit from services who do not meet the eligibility criteria. This is especially true of income-based services. Middle-class persons often find that they have too much income to be eligible for services from a government-funded agency, but too little income to feel comfortable paying the full cost of such services in the private sector. This is the one instance in which voluntary organizations can duplicate the services offered by community agencies: they duplicate the service but not the population served.

4. Voluntary organizations can focus their efforts on the development of caring relationships. Community agencies cannot afford to make caring (as defined in this volume) their primary mandate. They provide services, but they do not develop the kinds of relationships required for caring. Indeed, were the primary focus of voluntary organizations to be *caring,* they would never duplicate community agencies.

5. Voluntary organizations can offer care recipients more time than can community agencies. Agencies are under pressures to deliver services to as many people as possible at as little per capita cost as possible. These pressures result in a minimizing of time invested in individual recipients, albeit while providing the services most urgently needed. Voluntary organizations do not have to be under such time pressures. They can, for example, elect to serve no more care recipients than they have the capacity to serve without reducing the time needed to deliver those services effectively. Moreover, in developing caring relationships, considerably more time commitment is required than that involved in offering services.

6. Community agencies can seldom provide direct services to family caregivers (though services that directly benefit the impaired individual often indirectly benefit the caregiver as well). Although well aware of the emotional and physical costs that caregivers bear, the agencies typically must focus their energies on the needs of the ill or impaired person rather than the caregiver. Voluntary organizations, in contrast, can undertake both—caring not only for impaired individuals but also directly alleviating the suffering of caregivers.

Although voluntary organizations should, in my view, devote their energies to activities that do not compete with or duplicate those of community agencies, they also need to be realistic about what community agencies can do to help them. As noted previously, community agencies work under conditions of substantial constraints. All of the factors involved—

the specificity of their mandates, time, and financial resources—also constrain the extent to which they can assist voluntary organizations in establishing their programs, training their volunteers, and so forth. This is not a result of unwillingness to help but of their inability to do so. Community agencies are typically pleased to know about programs sponsored by voluntary organizations and to make them known to potential users. But this is likely to be the extent of their assistance.

THE INTERFACE BETWEEN VOLUNTARY ORGANIZATIONS AND INFORMAL SUPPORT SYSTEMS

At the same time that voluntary organizations develop and sustain an effective interface with community agencies, they also need to develop programs that take into account recipients' informal support systems. It is well established that friends and, especially, families are the cornerstone of both long-term care and caring in our society (see, e.g., Stone, 1987; Stone, Cafferata, and Sangl, 1987). They provide more assistance than any other source and they provide it for a longer period of time. Typically, there is a primary caregiver—generally the spouse or, in the absence of a spouse, an adult child. This primary person shoulders most of the caregiving responsibility and, as a consequence, is likely to experience substantial psychological distress (often, clinical depression) and perhaps physical health declines as well (see, e.g., George and Gwyther, 1986; Pruchno and Potashnik, 1989; Schulz and Williamson, 1991). In addition to providing the bulk of care, the primary caregiver also is the care receiver's staunchest ally and protector, defending as much as possible against unnecessary suffering, degradation, and assaults on the care receiver's dignity. Members of voluntary organizations who wish to benefit impaired persons need to recognize and plan their activities so that they mesh well with the concerns and issues of most concern to caregivers and other family members.

It must be understood that families typically need to retain control of the programs and volunteers who serve their impaired family members. If the impaired person is cognitively intact, he or she, too, will have a say in decisions concerning services, but even then the family typically serves as "gatekeeper," controlling access to the recipient. Impaired persons, whether cognitively intact or not, are seen by their loved ones as dependent and thus in need of unusual levels of protection.

Care programs—both formal service programs and those sponsored by voluntary organizations—underestimate the importance of this sense of control. Family members insist upon it. I can say this with confidence. A few years ago, we had a grant at Duke University to provide subsidized in-home respite care services to dementia patients in order to give their care-givers assistance, rest, and time free of caregiving responsibilities. To our surprise, very few caregivers agreed to use this service, even though it was free or very inexpensive (never more than $2 per hour) and utilized respite workers who were licensed nurses' aides, specifically trained to understand dementia. I interviewed a number of caregivers about the reasons for declining the respite care. I remember one woman, caring for her demented husband, who refused our respite care despite its being free. Instead, she preferred to continue paying an untrained "sitter" on an occasional basis. When I pointed out the advantages of our program, she replied, "I just feel like I'll have more control of how things are done if I'm the one who hires the sitter." This was an explicit statement of the caregivers' desire, or need, to retain control. Whatever services they offer, voluntary organizations must recognize this desire and work within its constraints. Simply offering appropriate free services is not enough.

Similarly, it is imperative that members of voluntary organizations develop relationships of trust with the primary caregiver and, in relevant cases, with other family members as well. Among the possible elements of developing such trust are putting up with the careful scrutiny of the caregiver until trust is established, assuring family members that all aspects of the interactions with the care recipient will be treated as confidential information, and assuring the caregiver that there is no implication in the offer of help that the care receiver is being treated inappropriately by family members. An especially touchy issue can be over comments made by a care receiver about family members. Care receivers need the opportunity to talk to persons other than family, and when, as it sometimes is, the talk is about family, this can be threatening to family members, who will often pump nonfamily care providers to hear what the care recipient said.

Under these conditions, the volunteer must strike a delicate balance between keeping the comments of the care recipient confidential and yet not angering the family. Voluntary organization members must keep in mind that securing trust is an ongoing matter; trust is not something obtained "once and for all."

For volunteer caregivers, reassuring family members that they are in control and earning their trust are challenges. But volunteers usually respond positively, desiring to forge a meaningful relationship with the care recipient and a caring partnership with family (Montgomery and Hatch,

1987). A frequent complaint caregivers voice about paid service providers or services delivered by agency personnel (public and private sector) is that they "really don't care" or are "just doing their jobs." If voluntary organization members can convince the caregiver that a caring relationship with the care receiver is the primary goal, with the provision of needed services being a means to that goal, the chances for success are greatly enhanced.

As noted above, a special quality of voluntary organizations is their ability to develop programs that are different from those offered by community agencies. This has important implications for securing the cooperation and trust of family caregivers. Many caregivers complain that agency services do not meet their needs. If they see that volunteers are willing and able to provide services that fit their needs, rather than those of the organization, they will be more receptive—and in all likelihood will benefit more from those services. For example, several caregivers have complained to me that, when dealing with agencies, services must be given at specific times and in specific amounts of time. If a caregiver desires respite on weekends or one evening a week, and home health aides are available only on weekdays, there is a mismatch between the caregiver's needs and the services available. Similarly, caregivers often would like to obtain an hour or so of assistance a day rather than receiving help in less-frequent four- or eight-hour blocks; for example, they might like help most days with bathing the care receiver. For obvious reasons, agencies cannot afford to send a home health aide for four one-hour trips rather than one four-hour trip; thus, the needs of the caregiver and care receiver cannot be met by the home health agency—an example of one of a myriad ways in which volunteers could step in. Putting the needs of the care receiver and caregiver first is a critical element of a caring relationship.

Programs offered by voluntary organizations also should be aware that care receivers' needs and abilities can change dramatically and quickly. Hopefully, volunteer programs can be designed to accommodate changes in needs without severing the relationship with the care receiver. A lack of such accommodation is a frequent complaint about community agencies. Frequently, if a care receiver's needs change (either lessening or increasing), that person is no longer eligible for services and the services are abruptly terminated. Part of a caring relationship is being there for the long haul and being responsive to changes in need. If voluntary organizations are to be successful in developing and sustaining caring relationships, they must be there for the long haul.

Finally, I will make explicit a theme implied throughout this section: caregivers need caring relationships, often as much as do the impaired persons for whom they care. Indeed, caregivers' needs are frequently (albeit often willingly) submerged because of the apparently greater needs of the impaired person. Community agencies recognize that caregivers need assistance, but typically they must focus primarily on the impaired person. As noted previously, community agencies are typically in the business of providing services, not that of developing caring relationships. Understanding the needs of caregivers and caring for them is an important contribution that can be made by voluntary organizations.

CONCLUSIONS AND FUTURE DIRECTIONS

Voluntary organizations can play a unique role in providing caring relationships to persons in need. Their greatest strengths are their flexibility and their ability to develop their own agendas, without the constraints faced by formal service programs of community agencies. Moreover, because they are flexible, voluntary organizations can make the development of caring relationships their first priority, with specific services serving as means to that end.

Two major obstacles, however, threaten the ability of voluntary organizations to foster caring relationships. First, the process of institutionalization often forces processes of bureaucratization that rival those of other organizations and/or require that most of an organization's effort be devoted to its own survival rather than to an agenda to serve others. Second, as I have argued here, in order to be effective in promoting caring relationships, members of voluntary organizations need to understand the issues that make their programs acceptable and valued by care receivers and their family members. It is not clear that these issues are widely understood and incorporated into the activities of voluntary organizations.

Another theme of this chapter is the need to honor the needs and values of the individual. This is, of course, an inherent component of caring. But true caring is rare, I think, and too often what is intended as caring ends up imposing the carer's values and agenda on the person in need. To refer briefly to my opening comments, a caring community, organization, or person will not smother the values of others or fail to respect an individual's needs as that person self-defines them.

I am, first and foremost, a researcher—albeit a caring one. I am disappointed at the extent to which this chapter was forced, as a result of lack of research findings, to rely on the implications of organizational theory and the substantial but anecdotal evidence that I have gathered from caregivers during the past fifteen years (my studies did not focus on the topic of this chapter). Research is desperately needed on many issues raised in this chapter: the desire of voluntary organizations to promote caring relationships, as compared with the less-difficult goal of sponsoring "service projects"; the conditions under which voluntary organizations are able to foster caring relationships; and the importance or lack thereof of the factors that I have suggested are essential for voluntary organizations to succeed in promoting caring relationships. We also need to determine the extent to which the four models described above—religious organizations, one-on-one programs, support groups, and caring communities—are differentially effective for specific populations (e.g., for nursing home residents, the homebound elderly, and the bereaved elderly). If one envisions the world of support and caring as divided into three sectors—formal agencies, informal support systems, and voluntary organizations—the latter is certainly the poor stepchild with regard to research evidence.

At the same time that I see a desperate need for research, we do not have to wait for that research to take place before encouraging voluntary organizations to contribute to caring for those who need it. They can be asked to do that now. Most importantly, perhaps, our whole society (in particular, members of voluntary organizations) needs to understand what caring is and the differences between caring relationships and the simpler provision of services or assistance. We do not have to wait for the research evidence to begin to educate the public about caring and encouraging individuals and organizations to commit themselves to it.

REFERENCES

Allport, G. W. (1950). *The Individual and His Religion: A Psychological Interpretation.* New York: Macmillan.

Cohen, C. I., Hyland, K., and Devlin, M. (1999). An evaluation of the use of the natural helping network model to enhance the well-being of nursing home residents. *Gerontologist* 39: 426–33.

Curtis, J. E., Grabb, E., and Baer, D. (1992). Voluntary association membership in fifteen countries. *American Sociological Review* 57: 137–52.

de Tocqueville, A. ([1835] 1956). *Democracy in America.* New York: Mentor.

DiMaggio, P. J., and Powell, W. W. (1983). The iron cage revisited: Institutional isomorphism and collective rationality in organizational fields. *American Sociological Review* 48: 147–60.

George, L. K., and Gwyther, L. P. (1986). Caregiver well-being: A multidimensional examination of family caregivers of demented adults. *Gerontologist* 26: 253–59.
Greene, V. L., and Monahan, D. J. (1989). The effect of a support and education program on stress and burden among family caregivers to frail elderly persons. *Gerontologist* 29: 472–77.
Halpert, B. P. (1988). Volunteer information provider program: A strategy to reach and help rural family caregivers. *Gerontologist:* 28: 256–59.
Hochschild, A. R. (1973). *The Unexpected Community.* Berkeley: University of California Press.
Kanter, R. M. (1972). *Commitment and Community: Communes and Utopias in Sociological Perspective.* Cambridge: Harvard University Press.
Levy, L. H., Derby, J. F., and Martinkowski, K. S. (1993). Effects of membership in bereavement support groups on adaptation to conjugal bereavement. *American Journal of Community Psychology* 21: 361–81.
Lieberman, M. A., Borman, L. D., and Associates (1979). *Self-Help Groups for Coping with Crisis.* San Francisco: Jossey-Bass.
Luks, A., and Payne, P. (1992). *The Healing Power of Doing Good: The Health and Spiritual Benefits of Helping Others.* New York: Fawcett Columbine.
Matthews, S. H. (1979). *The Social World of Old Women.* Beverly Hills, CA: Sage.
McMillan, D. W., and Chavis, D. M. (1986). Sense of community: A definition and theory. *Journal of Community Psychology* 14: 6–23.
Montgomery, R. J. V., and Hatch, L. R. (1987). The feasibility of volunteers and families forming a partnership for caregiving. In T. H. Brubaker, ed., *Aging, Health, and Family,* pp. 75–92. Beverly Hills, CA: Sage.
Murnigham, J. K., Kim, J. W., and Metzer, A. R. (1993). The volunteer dilemma. *Administrative Science Quarterly* 38: 515–38.
Omoto, A. M., and Snyder, M. (1995). Sustained helping without obligation: Motivation, longevity, and perceived attitude change among AIDS volunteers. *Journal of Personality and Social Psychology* 68: 671–86.
Pancoast, D. L., Parker, P., and Froland, C. (1983). *Rediscovering Self-Help: Its Role in Social Care.* Beverly Hills, CA: Sage.
Piliavin, J. A., and Charng, H. W. (1990). Altruism: A review of recent theory and research. *Annual Review of Sociology* 16: 27–65.
Powell, W. W. (1985). The institutionalization of rational organizations. *Contemporary Sociology* 14: 564–66.
Pruchno, R. A., and Potashnik, S. L. (1989). Caregiving spouses: Physical and mental health in perspective. *Journal of the American Geriatrics Society* 37: 697–705.
Rubinstein, R. L. (1986). *Singular Paths: Old Men Living Alone.* New York: Columbia University Press.
Sarason, S. B. (1976). *The Psychological Sense of Community: Prospects for a Community Psychology.* San Francisco: Jossey-Bass.

Schulz, R., and Williamson, G. M. (1991). A 2-year longitudinal study of depression among Alzheimer caregivers. *Psychology and Aging* 6: 569–78.

Scott, W. R. (1995). *Institutions and Organizations.* Thousand Oaks, CA: Sage.

Silverman, P. R. (1980). *Mutual Help Groups: Organization and Development.* New York: Springer Publishing.

Skirboll, B., and Pavelsky, P. (1984). The Compeer program: Volunteers as friends of the mentally ill. *Hospital and Community Psychiatry* 35: 938–39.

Stack, C. B. (1974). *All Our Kin: Strategies for Survival in the Black Community.* New York: Harper & Row.

Stone, R. (1987). *Exploding the Myths: Caregiving in America: A Study.* Washington, DC: U.S. Congress, House Select Committee on Aging.

Stone, R., Cafferata, G., and Sangl, J. (1987). Caregivers of the frail elderly: A national profile. *Gerontologist* 30: 616–26.

Thompson, J. D. (1967). *Organizations in Action.* New York: McGraw Hill.

Tomasi, L., ed. (1998). *The Tradition of the Chicago School of Sociology.* Brookfield, VT: Ashgate.

Toseland, R., Rossiter, C., and Labrecque, M. (1989). The effectiveness of two kinds of support groups for caregivers. *Social Service Review* 63: 415–32.

Webster's New Universal Unabridged Dictionary. 2nd ed. (1979). New York: Simon & Schuster.

Wilson, J., and Janowski, T. (1995). The contribution of religion to volunteer work. *Sociology of Religion* 56: 137–52.

Zucker, L., ed. (1988). *Institutional Patterns and Organizations: Culture and Environment.* Cambridge, MA: Bollinger.

III

ASSESSMENTS OF CARING

10

Appraising the Success of Caring

ALVAN R. FEINSTEIN, M.D.

APPRAISING the quality of medical care has been a dynamically growing activity for the past three decades. Although efforts to evaluate and improve care were made by Florence Nightingale (Nightingale, 1863) in the nineteenth century and by Ernest A. Codman (Codman, 1917 [1996]) early in the twentieth, the recent growth in the United States has been spurred by financial incentives. The federal government, commercial organizations (such as insurance companies), and private foundations have all sought to reduce the increasing costs of care while hoping to maintain satisfactory quality.

The incentives offered by these groups have spawned a large array of organizations and programs that have struggled with the challenges of deciding what to regard as quality of care, choosing ways to measure it, and developing improved mechanisms to deliver it. The challenges have been complex and difficult because quality is like both beauty and pornography: like beauty, it is often in the eye of the beholder; like pornography, it is often hard to define but easy to recognize.

My goal in this chapter is to indicate that the total activities of *care* contain elements of *curing* and *caring;* but almost all existing procedures for appraising "quality of care" today are aimed only at curing. Because the existing procedures cannot adequately evaluate caring, a new approach is proposed at the end of the chapter.

DIVERSION OF GOALS AND CONCEPTS

Efforts to define quality of care have frequently used the "avoid-and-divert" policy that is common in modern medical science. For example, the search for a suitable definition of excellent clinicians has often been diverted to the demand that they pass an appropriate certifying examination. Analogously, the question of what to regard as quality of care has usually been avoided by diverting the response to answers available from diverse measurements and mechanisms of health care delivery. Thus, the easily measured rates of mortality or postoperative complications have often been used to indicate the quality of surgical procedures; and the easily ascertained existence of appropriate facilities and numbers of personnel has denoted the quality of a hospital or other health care system.

This avoid-and-divert strategy is not new or unusual. For most of the twentieth century, as individuals, groups, and societies have been both benefited and harmed by the impact of magnificent technology, investigators in the social, behavioral, and clinical sciences have generally preferred an exact answer to a diverted question rather than an imprecise or approximate answer to the direct question. More than fifty years ago, the strategy was summarized for the social sciences in Frank Knight's memorable aphorism: "If you cannot measure, measure anyhow" (Wirth, 1940: 169).

Perhaps the most obvious diversion has been the altered concept of the word *care* itself. The traditional medical idea is that care denotes concern, empathy, compassion, and other Samaritan aspects of the doctor's attitude toward the patient (McDermott and Rogers, 1983). Today, however, particularly as doctors have come to be called providers, *care* usually refers to the array of activities performed by providers in "managing" the patients, who are often called consumers. The interpersonal activities once called care are now usually called caring, and the phenomena subsumed as care generally refer to entities that might best be called curing.

The change in terms from *doctors* to *providers* is not unreasonable, since many persons other than physicians regularly contribute to the activities of care. The use of *care* to refer to management rather than caring is also not unreasonable, since *care* is probably the best simple word for denoting the total scope of activities in preventing or treating disease.

The word *disease* has also changed, of course. Before the nineteenth century, it referred to a patient's discomforted ease—that is, *dis-ease*—but it now denotes a more abstract entity, often manifested by morphologic or laboratory abnormalities that were not discernible before the advent of modern technology. (The symptoms and other direct clinical manifestations that were once called dis-ease are now usually cited as illness.) Even the change from *patient* to *consumer* is also defensible since *patient* comes from the Latin, *pati,* which means "to suffer"; and not all persons receiving care

are in a state of suffering. Nevertheless, the many changes in nomenclature and usage reflect the profound alterations of a long-standing medical tradition. A suffering patient who received caring has been replaced by a consumer whose diseases are to be cured by preventive or remedial management. The activities of that management are what become appraised today as *quality of care.* The appraisal procedures might be criticized for not reflecting the goal of caring, but they are a product (and reflection) of major changes that had occurred in the world of medical "care" long before the appraisal procedures were developed.

DOMAINS OF QUALITY OF CARE

To facilitate measurement, quality of care has been divided into different domains that might be cataloged as components, constituents, and standard setting, and that are approached with different methods for expressing and evaluating the contents of the domains. An early and now often-used approach was proposed when Donabedian (1980, 1982) divided the domains of quality of care into three main components. The components could then be subdivided into diverse constituents; and standards could be set for evaluating the constituents.

Components

Donabedian's three main components were called structure, process, and outcome. *Structure* refers to the personnel, facilities, and system involved in health care delivery. *Process* refers to the actions that emerge from those structural elements. *Outcome* denotes the subsequent events that follow the process. For example, a nurse practitioner (as part of structure) might recommend (as part of process) an analgesic for the treatment of headache. As outcome, the headache might or might not be relieved.

This classification produced an excellent basic taxonomy for demarcating the entities to be considered, but an immediate problem was apparent. The three sets of entities occurred sequentially, but were not consequential. Effects could not always be attributed to or associated with the antecedent "causes." Thus, when a factory manufactures inanimate objects, an excellent structure and process should always be followed by an excellent outcome. In the vicissitudes of the medical ailments and personal interchanges of human life, however, a good structure may be accompanied by a poor process, and vice versa. Furthermore, a good outcome may occur despite inadequacies in both structure and process; and a splendid structure and process may sometimes be followed by a poor outcome. For example, my great-grandmother delivered nine healthy babies at home (or in a farm field) without any special prenatal care or medical attendance. Conversely, a stillbirth can occasionally occur today despite excellent "care" during the pregnancy, accompanied by multiple sonograms, superb hospital facilities, and a board-certified obstetrician.

Because of the dissociations and uncertainties, an unresolved conflict has existed about where to focus the main evaluation of quality of care. On one side are those who argue that only outcomes are important; on the other side is the argument that only structure and process can be really improved because outcomes are too dependent on unalterable (and often unpredictable) biologic phenomena of disease and human beings. What are often ignored during the argument, however, are the different constituents of structure, process, and outcome, and the interrelationships among those constituents.

Constituents

Each of the three component domains contains constituent entities that have both form and function. The forms can usually be easily identified, specified, and documented. Thus, in a particular health care system, we can count such structural elements as the number of registered nurses, board-certified doctors, and transportation orderlies, and the existence of a hospital ombudsman for patients' complaints. For a specified clinical condition, we can document whether an inappropriate treatment was used, or whether an appropriate treatment was omitted or given at the right time. To address the form of an outcome, we can identify whether the patient survived, whether blood pressure or blood lipids were reduced, and whether a low hematocrit was raised.

The form of each of these constituent entities, however, is accompanied by behavioral and functional phenomena that are more difficult to measure. Are the nurses and doctors empathic and compassionate? Do the transportation orderlies take patients to a radiologic suite and then abandon them in the hallway? Is the ombudsman merely a titular position or is it someone who is truly available, empowered to act, and able to evoke appropriate remedial actions?

When pursuing the form of the orders placed for appropriate (or inappropriate) diagnostic tests and treatments, do the hospital personnel suitably explain their decisions and prepare the patients for what is going to happen? Is the form of the outcome entities restricted to survival and easily obtained technologic measurements, or do they include such functions as the patient's anxiety, discomfort, physical capacity, and satisfaction with care?

These behavioral and functional phenomena are much more difficult to measure than the existence and dimensions of form for constituent elements. Consequently, the functional phenomena are seldom measured, and, when "measured," are seldom checked for personal interrelationships. Accordingly, the close correlation that might occur between certain processes and outcomes is seldom documented; and the discussion may be relegated to the scientifically disreputable status of anecdotes. For example, although death may be counted as a poor outcome despite appropriate therapy, the patient's serenity and the family's tranquility during the period of dying may be an excellent outcome that can be directly associated with thoughtful, compassionate care by the medical and nursing staff. The anecdotes may also include many instances in which a disgruntled patient and family took legal action against an arrogant surgeon, despite an apparently good outcome, and yet other instances in which a patient and family, happy about sensitive attention from the health care system and personnel, did not seek legal redress for gross errors in therapy.

The form/function distinction in the constituent elements also reflects the difference between caring and curing. The elements of form in the existence or dimensions of specified constituents are usually measured in reference to such curing outcomes as survival and restoration of physiologic normality. The functional performance of the elements, however, is seldom examined for their contributions to such caring outcomes as serenity, tranquillity, and good quality of life. Consequently, the possibility that caring outcomes might be highly correlated with structure and process is usually missed when the correlation measurements are restricted solely to outcomes aimed at curing.

Standards of Evaluation

Setting standards of evaluation is often regarded as the most difficult part of appraising quality of care, not just because the necessary information may be omitted from collection, but particularly because of disagreements about how the standards should be set and applied. The topics that give rise to these disagreements can be divided into two main parts: ideologic disputes and methodologic problems in statistical expressions. The topics are extensive enough to warrant separate discussion in the next few sections.

IDEOLOGIC DISPUTES

The disputes labeled here as *ideologic* arise from ideas or doctrines that cannot be documented as proved. They represent beliefs and preferences, such as choice of vocation, avocation, religion, political party, or type of entertainment. Each set of preferences can be accompanied by its own justifications and rationales, and each choice may be worthwhile or self-defeating, defensible or attackable. The choices themselves, however, cannot be demonstrated as either right or wrong, although the decisions can profoundly affect the way a person lives, enjoys life, and dies.

In the field of quality of care, the ideologic decisions arise from the choice of viewpoints, criteria, scope, and grading of the evaluations.

Viewpoints

Whose viewpoint should be used when quality of care is evaluated? For sociologists and economists, the view is usually aimed at society or systems of health care. This view is encouraged by national organizations that are concerned with public expenditures, corporate profits, or such general goals as universal access to care.

The clinical and public health investigators who examine quality of care, however, usually work at (or get data from) a particular institution. They often know the associated health care personnel and may enlist them in consultation or collaboration. The research activities may then use the viewpoint of the professional personnel.

A third viewpoint is that of the individual persons who receive the care. This viewpoint might seem appropriate and desirable, but is seldom used. The main argument against it is that most patients are regarded as not qualified to make decisions about the efficiency of a system, the competence of the personnel, the appropriateness of therapy, or the appraisal of a clinical outcome. Besides, many patients may be too subjective, inconsistent, or nonrational to make delicate judgments. (Very little evidence exists, however, to demonstrate that patients are necessarily more subjective, inconsistent, and nonrational than the concomitant health care personnel.)

The omission of the patient's viewpoint may seem to make things more scientific, but it also tends to make curing rather than caring the main focus of evaluation. The system and the professional staff can readily use their background knowledge and foreground goals to examine curative phenomena; but caring is usually best discerned by its recipients.

An additional problem is that many acts of caring are difficult or complex to describe; and they are seldom entered in the medical records from which care is often evaluated. An arm across the shoulder, a hug, a squeeze of the hand, a subtle perception, a compassionate response, a useful explanation, a thoughtful comment to the patients' spouse or child, a rearrangement of the bedclothes, an appropriate drawing of curtains or lowering of voice—these can all be important acts of caring. Nevertheless, unlike the "curative" data of laboratory and technologic procedures, the information about these elements of caring is seldom entered in the medical record. Having devoted the extra time to do the caring, its provider may not want to take additional time to record the details. Furthermore, in some of the new-style computerized medical records, which allegedly save time (i.e., allow more time for acts of caring), no format may be available to report them, even if the provider wants to do so.

Criteria

Separate topics of dispute are the approach used for setting criteria, and the choice of the standards to be applied in grading.

To evaluate care for a particular patient, we would need to consider everything that happened: the presenting manifestations, the first set of clinical decisions (often a diagnostic work-up), the next set of clinical decisions (often a choice of consultation or therapy), and all the subsequent decisions, actions, and events. Because each patient's situation will usually have its own individual distinctions, standard criteria could not be developed for routine application to all possible cases. The appraisal of each patient's care could still be done, however, if suitable expert appraisers review what happened and apply their own implicit criteria and standards during the evaluation. (This type of evaluation also occurs during the oral examination of a candidate for board certification or for higher academic degrees.)

The use of implicit criteria has the advantage of being aimed at the right thing—the total care of a patient—but it is associated with many scientific disadvantages. The appraisers who do the work may not always be suitable in skill, temperament, objectivity, and consistency. In the absence of specifications for the criteria, the different appraisers may reach different decisions for the same case; and whatever is learned during the evaluation process cannot be identified and cited for justification or for application elsewhere.

To obtain the detailed specifications needed for *ex*plicit criteria, however, the scope of evaluation must be sharply narrowed. Instead of checking an unselected series of patients, the appraisers may check a highly selected set of tracer, or indicator, conditions (Kessler, Kalk, and Singer, 1973) that are reasonably common and important in a large group of patients. In primary-care practice, for example, these conditions might include sore throat, urinary tract symptoms, back pain, and hypertension. In a consultant or hospital practice, the conditions might include acute myocardial infarction and acute gastrointestinal bleeding. After the tracer conditions have been selected, explicit criteria can be constructed and applied to appraise the management of each condition. (In a modern extension of the activity, such criteria are now prepared and offered not just for retrospective evaluation of care, but particularly for prospective instructions to the providers. The new criteria are called guidelines, or critical pathways.)

Scope

Explicit criteria have the obvious scientific virtues of being stipulated, up front, and applicable by diverse evaluators, not just by experts. On the other hand, the criteria pertain only to the selected conditions and are often applied, despite all the detailed explications, with substantial inter-rater variations (Goldman, 1992). Perhaps the greatest disadvantage, however, is in scope. The specifications in the criteria are almost always aimed at acts of testing, ordering, and performance that can easily be determined in the medical record. Consequently, the explicit criteria become yet another mechanism for emphasizing activities of curing rather than caring.

This same disadvantage, of course, occurs with implicit criteria, since the main source of the difficulty is the use of medical records, which seldom contain the information needed for the evaluations. Nevertheless, an expert who appraises the patient's entire record, rather than just the segment needed for management of the tracer condition, may sometimes find acts of caring mentioned in nurses' notes, clinical progress notes, or other locations (for many medical records, the expert appraiser must first be able to master the formidable challenge of reading handwriting before making any additional discernments). In such sites as office practices, nursing homes, or hospices, however, the medical records often have a much more limited set of entries; and for patients treated at home, no record may be available.

For all these reasons, caring (rather than curing) cannot be evaluated from information recorded by the providers of care. The evaluation procedure for caring must either contain direct observation and monitoring or must rely on retrospective inquiry from recipients. Direct observation is expensive and time-intensive; and retrospective inquiry and subjective reports will raise hackles in the scientific community.

Standards and Grading

The fourth set of ideologic issues refers to the setting of standards and grading of the evaluations.

Before the standards are set for evaluating care, decisions must be made about what to evaluate. Should each case be checked in an individual, unselected manner or should there be a focus on patients with "tracer conditions"? If the latter, which conditions should be chosen? For either unselected cases or tracer conditions, should the entire course of care be reviewed or should it be only individual episodes? For example, if a patient has recurrent episodes of congestive heart failure or asthma attacks, the care given between episodes may sometimes be more important than what is used for each episode. For a patient with persistent chronic conditions such as hemiplegia, urinary incontinence, or dementia, the criteria and evaluation procedure will be quite different from what is pertinent for asymptomatic hypertension, diabetes mellitus, or hyperlipidemia. Furthermore, although most of the efforts devoted to setting standards have been aimed at curative topics, issues in caring are particularly pertinent for patients with permanent disabilities or with ongoing impairment in activities of daily living.

Assuming that these decisions about what to evaluate have been satisfactory, we can then proceed to the standards used for the evaluation. When acts of care are deemed appropriate or inappropriate, excellent or poor, laudable or reprehensible, who should choose the grades used for the ratings and the standards that elicit a rating for each grade?

Should the standard setters be expert consultants? Ordinary practitioners? Nurses? Economists? Or the members of the public who receive the care? Elitist standards set by expert consultants at tertiary care institutions may be appropriate for those institutions but unsuitable for the work of representative practitioners elsewhere. For example, during my six-year term as a member of the governing group of the American Board of Internal Medicine, I not once succeeded in getting the written examination to include a question for which the answer was "do nothing" or "watchful waiting." Although proposed as a response to several clinical scenarios, this answer was unacceptable to many of my specialist colleagues in the committee. In each scenario, they regularly found something they would do.

An effective way of choosing the standard setters might be to focus on the entity being evaluated. If it represents a curative action, the standard might be set by persons most appropriate to evaluate the merits of the action and its pertinence in different clinical situations and locations. If the action is related to cost-efficiency ratios, the decisions might be made by economists or a clinicoeconomic collaboration. If the entity is a caring phenomenon, however, the standards might be best set by patients and family, perhaps aided by skilled nurses.

Regardless of who sets the standards, their role requires separate consideration. Are they intended to give general grades to all acts of care and perhaps to elevate the average performance of care? Or are they supposed to detect the outlier providers who are particularly poor performers (an activity sometimes called "getting the dangerous drivers off the road")? If the goal is to find and perhaps improve or remove the undesirable outliers, the standards might be set in a simple pass/fail manner according to egregiously unacceptable performance of certain critical challenges.

For example, analgesics for an ordinary tension headache might be regarded as an appropriate recommendation in ordinary primary care, but some other mechanisms of relief (such as rest or whiskey) might not be greatly downgraded or deemed grossly inappropriate. Consultation with a neurologist, and particularly with a neurosurgeon, however, might be regarded as an outlying, improper decision. On the other hand, suppose the patient has had recurrent tension headaches, is emotionally alarmed about them, and insists on more elaborate care? Is the doctor then remiss in ordering a brain scan or an expert consultation?

Finally, the last challenge to be cited in setting standards is the external problem of whether sins of commission are more serious than those of omission. In the old, pretechnology medical era, the guiding principle was *primum non nocere* (above all, do no harm). Today, however, with so many powerful but sometimes harmful agents available, the doctor who always seeks to avoid harm will also fail to provide important benefits. A more frequent guiding principle today, therefore, is to seek an optimum risk/benefit ratio. Nevertheless, what may be deemed an appropriate omission may sometimes lead to adverse effects, and sins of commission may sometimes have major benefits. For example, giving antibiotics for the common cold is usually condemned as grossly inappropriate. On the other hand, in patients who apparently have a common cold, many Group A streptococcal infections can exist without producing the classical manifestations of pharyngitis and can be successfully treated by the antibiotic. In fact, the virtual disappearance of acute rheumatic fever in the United States is often ascribed to the overuse of antibiotics that were given for the common cold but that, incidentally, eradicated many potentially noxious streptococci. The practitioner who does not give the antibiotic may be lauded, but the acclaim may not be shared by the rare patient whose untreated streptococcal infection leads to rheumatic fever or glomerulonephritis.

On the other hand, a doctor may get full credit for excellent practice in the sphere of curing if a patient with acute myocardial infarction is admitted to an intensive care unit, monitored with all the pertinent equipment, and given all the appropriate medication while in the hospital and at discharge. The doctor may not, however, have offered any words of caring assurance while the patient was terrified by associated events in the intensive care unit, and may not do so later when the patient is at home after discharge, an invalid, fearing death at any moment.

STATISTICAL METHODS

Another reason for diverting quality-of-care assessments to topics of curing rather than caring is that curing can much more easily be cited in terms currently amenable to quantitative statistical expressions. The use of statistics in medicine, rudimentary when the twentieth century began, has now become a customary and often dominant activity. The quality of a nation's health care is often rated according to statistical data for longevity and infant mortality rates. A hospital's quality of care may be cited according to mortality rates and counts of personnel and equipment. New drugs will be licensed only if accompanied by "statistically significant" data from randomized clinical trials; and meta-analytic statistical aggregations of randomized-trial data have become the basis for what is now called evidence-based medicine. The considerable benefits produced by the statistical activities are well recognized and beyond dispute, but like all other potent interventions, they have had many adverse side effects.

Humanists often complain that modern medicine has become too oriented toward reductionist science. To explain mechanisms of disease and human biology, the scientific methods have progressively reduced the investigated entities downward from intact organisms to organs and systems, then to tissues and fluids, and ultimately to membranes, cells, and molecules. Since the study of intact people is essentially eliminated in this approach, reductionist medical science is often accused of being dehumanized.

On the other hand, the reductionist approach is entirely appropriate for the goal of exploring mechanisms of biologic action, and the approach has led to magnificent scientific advances in technology, in therapy, and in understanding diverse mechanisms of development for human ailments. What is often overlooked during the attack on biologic reductionism is the much greater antihumanistic threat of statistical reductionism by researchers who are apparently studying patient care.

Statistical reductionism—as discussed in the next few sections—occurs with mathematical or psychometric methods that (1) rely on "hard" data, avoiding the crucial "soft" data of distress and caring; (2) express complex phenomena not as a coordinated whole but as an aggregate of multiple items; (3) purposely ask questions in a general, depersonalized manner; (4) deliberately eliminate important personal details; and (5) report results for an "average" person.

Reliance on Hard Data

Most studies of therapy have relied on outcome events delineated by so-called hard data, such as death, diagnoses of disease, and laboratory or morphologic data. The statisticians are justified in wanting to use "reliable" data and avoid the soft information of symptoms, patterns of illness, and other crucial personal phenomena. The focus on hard data, however, helps produce a dehumanized set of information and also allows clinical personnel to continue avoiding the challenge of making the soft data respectable. The respectability could easily be attained if clinicians acknowledged the importance of the challenge and then worked to improve the methods of observing and expressing the pertinent phenomena. A pioneer in this type of clinimetric approach almost fifty years ago was Virginia Apgar, who converted the implicit rating of a newborn baby's condition into the explicit score by which she is commemorated (Apgar, 1953).

Getting a Whole from Aggregated Parts

The Apgar score converted a so-called soft rating for a whole phenomenon, such as excellent for a newborn baby's condition, to a relatively hard aggregated sum of five parts (or items), each rated as 0, 1, or 2. The approach was successful because she chose the five parts according to sensible clinical judgment about importance; and the score she produced was easy to remember and to use.

The same strategy seems to have been applied in statistical and psychometric methods that also produce the rating for a whole from a sum of aggregated parts. The results appear in multivariable analyses that predict complex phenomena, such as prognosis, by using such aggregated mathematical sums as $Y = b_1X_1 + b_2X_2 + b_3X_3 + b_4X_4 + \ldots$, where the X values represent individual variables, and the b values are coefficients for the weights of each variable. The results also appear when other complex phenomena such as satisfaction with care, functional status, or quality of life are indexed as the sum of ratings for a series of multiple items that are regarded as constituents of the phenomena.

Although seemingly similar to Apgar's basic strategy, the statistical and psychometric methods are carried out with striking clinical differences (Feinstein, 1999). Apgar chose a small number of crucial variables, using the "dissected intuition" of her clinical experience. The mathematical methods employ a much larger number of variables—usually thirty or more; their importance is determined not with clinical judgment but from mathematical calculations; and the variables often do not include crucial phenomena, such as clinical severity and comorbidity for prognosis, or spirituality and emotional satisfaction for quality of life. Apgar took a carefully considered whole and suitably demarcated its parts. The mathematical methods, after aggregating a set of arbitrarily chosen and arbitrarily weighted parts, claim that their sum is a rating for the whole.

Clinicians have traditionally used the Apgarian clinimetric approach when they asked the questions "How are you?" and then asked further questions such as "In what way?" or "What bothers you the most?" This approach has often been dismissed, however, as lacking the statistical credentials of reliability and validity. The substitute mathematical approach is conducted essentially as "Please enter your responses to this lengthy set of questions, and then I will tell you how you are."

The conversion of a complex whole to a set of aggregated parts is the essence of reductionism; it is, however, often employed for such humanistic goals as determining satisfaction with care or quality of life. Since the procedure usually deprives patients of stating their own distinctive desires, expectations, and discontents, the failure to develop and apply a better technique is yet another manifestation of the avoid-and-divert phenomenon.

Depersonalized Questions

Another problem in the psychometric approach is the reluctance to ask direct questions (Feinstein, 1987). The direct approach might say, "Do you like your doctor? If not, why not?"; the psychometric tactic, on the other hand, might have responses ranging from strongly agree to strongly disagree for statements such as "Most people like their doctors" and "Most doctors carefully explain and report results for the tests they have ordered." The information may receive satisfactory statistical credentials, but it may not lend itself to separating out patients' attitudes toward their personal doctors from their feelings about doctors in general; in this regard, interpretation may be impossible.

The Elimination of Important Personal Details

The essence of statistical analysis is the reduction and elimination of details. A simple example is the use of "three significant digits" to express the value of π; i.e., as 3.14, rather than 3.14159 . . . . A more compelling example is the reduction of a distribution of data to a single central index, such as the mean, or median. The reductionism can be highly valuable when applied to the decimal digits of a number or to offer the "univariate" summary value for a single variable, such as age, weight, or blood pressure. The reductionism is undesirable, however, when it eliminates variables rather than digits or distributions. A thoughtful caregiver—who will consider the patients' age and weight and blood pressure and a great many other variables such as disability, distress, and social support—is not well served by results that not only eliminate the latter three variables but may not even include them in the collected data.

The Use of "Average" Results

The reduction of detail is a reasonable, necessary part of statistical analysis. No analyses could be done if all of a person's individual details were always considered. Unless the details are reduced enough to allow suitable groups to be delineated, the groups will be too small for their membership to contain reasonably stable numbers that can be attributable to factors other than chance probabilities alone. Thus, if we want "statistically significant" results, we need big groups, but to get big groups, we must reduce the descriptive detail for each group.

This conflict produces another major dilemma in modern medical care. During the past half century, the use of randomized clinical trials has led to majestic advances in therapeutic science. In contrast to the anecdotes, authoritarian doctrines, and unquantified clinical judgments of the past, documentary evidence has become available, for the first time in medical history, to demonstrate the efficacy of therapeutic agents. The patients admitted to the trials, however, may all have the same basic clinical condition or disease being treated, but may be otherwise heterogeneous in having diverse personal and pathophysiologic characteristics.

The randomization process may distribute those diverse characteristics in an equitable manner among the compared therapeutic groups, but the final results pertain to an average patient in each group. These average results have been splendid for the overall decisions made by regulatory agencies, pharmaceutical manufacturers, and other general evaluators of therapeutic efficacy. The results have also been valuable when efficacious agents were chosen for cost-benefit and cost-effectiveness analysis and when "guidelines" and "critical pathways" were established for general policy decisions in clinical practice.

The average results of randomized clinical trials, however, have not been satisfactory for clinical decisions about the care of individual patients. To demonstrate efficacy, a particular therapeutic agent may have been compared against placebo, not against other effective agents; and the trial data may not contain (or report) adequate information for the patients' distinctive clinical and demographic subgroups. Like other major scientific and statistical advances, the average results may be excellent for public policy decisions, but not for individual decisions about patient care.

ACHIEVING MEASUREMENTS AND STANDARDS FOR CARING

For all of the foregoing reasons, the procedures that have been developed for measuring quality of care cannot be satisfactory for appraising success in caring. If such appraisals are desired, a new set of procedures will be needed. They can probably best be developed not by delegating the task to outside methodologists and other external consultants, but by persons who are intimately familiar with what actually occurs; that is, who know the needs and activities of caring. Those persons will be patients, caregivers, family members, and associated contributors, rather than more distant medical personnel.

A first step would be to ask the pertinent participants for particularly bad or good examples of caring. The questions should be asked in an open-ended manner, allowing a free range of topics and scope of comments in the responses. The examples that are mentioned should be reported not in general phrases such as "thoughtless," "communicates well," or "insensitive," but in specific descriptions such as "abandoned me in the hall outside the radiology suite," "told me exactly what to expect when I went for the MRI," or "was unaware of the religious and cultural anxiety of a devout Catholic admitted to a Jewish hospital."

When enough specific examples have been accumulated, they can be organized into the more general categories of an appropriate taxonomy. Such a tactic was used to construct the taxonomic categories when Matthews and Feinstein (1988) prepared a "review of systems for the personal aspects of patient care" in a hospital, and when the taxonomy was later applied by patients to rate physicians' performance in a hospital setting (Matthews and Feinstein, 1989).

The procedure may lead to a multi-item inventory that at first resembles the multiple items used in psychometric strategies. The inventory of caring, however, will have several major differences. The items will have been chosen, for both topics and importance, by the respondents, rather than by the investigators or by a mathematical rating system. The performance of the individual cited entities may be given simple binary ratings (*yes/no* or *present/absent*) rather than ordinal categories (such as *strongly agree, strongly disagree*) or ordinal frequencies (such as *always, often, never*). And the results can be used not to achieve an aggregated score of points but to denote individual problems that need solutions. In addition, the inventory itself can offer powerful details of phenomena to be considered when caring is taught or evaluated.

However, the current challenges in caring for patients with chronic illness, permanent disabilities, and premoribund conditions will require more extensive information than that obtained for hospital situations. The work will need input not just from patients but also from families, caregivers, and other pertinent persons. The standard constituents used for structure in Donabedian's classification will also need expansion to include nursing homes, assisted-living facilities, adult day care centers, hospices, and other sites where caring occurs. The constituents should also include other participating personnel (nurses' aides, visiting nurses, physical and occupational therapists, clergy, social workers, family members, close friends, volunteers) beyond doctors, nurses, and administrators.

After all the elements of caring have been identified, the criteria for "successful" caring should be established by recipients and the other participants; they are the people most appropriate for determining what is needed and wanted and for appraising how well the hopes and desires are fulfilled. The work of identifying the elements and establishing criteria can be greatly aided by assistance from a capable methodologist and a knowledgeable clinician, who could help decide whether realistic goals are being set. The methodologist, however, should come with an open mind, prepared to discover reality, learn from it, and develop appropriate new ways to analyze it. The project can be greatly harmed rather than helped if the methodologist arrives with preconceived notions and rigid principles of conventional statistical or psychometric doctrines.

The challenges in such a project are new, having been inadequately approached by the methods of the past. Accordingly, the methods needed to master the new challenges will require new viewpoints and approaches. The same dimensional measurements used for a volume of urine, milligrams of sodium, or duration of survival will never be applicable for appraising acts of communication, compassion, or help. For people who believe these acts are worthwhile and important, however, they can easily be recognized, identified, classified, and organized into an effective taxonomy. About a century ago, believing that chemistry was an artful but important entity, Mendeleyev constructed a fundamental taxonomy called the periodic table. His job was relatively easy because he needed to consider only two constituents: weight and valence. The result, however, was an essential basis for all the subsequent scientific progress that has now led to modern technology, with its magnificent achievements and sometimes lamentable consequences in humane medicine and in caring for patients.

Although caring is one of the oldest activities of human existence and medical practice, the procedures of caring have now become extraordinarily challenging, because they have been omitted not only from the education given to most modern physicians but also from the customary appraisals of "care." Since the art of caring is well known to the people who give and receive it, the main challenge now is to identify, appraise, and teach the constituents of the art. It need not be made into a science per se, but an appropriate taxonomy of constituents can provide new dignity, respect, attention, and development.

REFERENCES

Apgar, V. (1953). A proposal for a new method of evaluation of the newborn infant. *Anesthesia and Analgesia* 32: 260–67.

Codman, E. A. (1917 [1996]). *A Study in Hospital Efficiency.* Privately printed; reprint, Oakbrook, IL: Joint Commission on Accreditation of Healthcare Organizations.

Donabedian, A. (1980). *Explorations in Quality Assessment and Monitoring:* 1, *Definition of Quality and Approaches to Its Assessment.* Ann Arbor, MI: Health Administration Press.

Donabedian, A. (1982). *Explorations in Quality Assessment and Monitoring:* 2, *The Criteria and Standards of Quality.* Ann Arbor, MI: Health Administration Press.

Feinstein, A. R. (1987). *Clinimetrics.* New Haven, CT: Yale University Press.

Feinstein, A. R. (1999). Multi-item "instruments" vs. Virginia Apgar's principles of clinimetrics. *Archives of Internal Medicine* 159: 125–28.

Goldman, R. L. (1992). The reliability of peer assessments of quality of care. *Journal of the American Medical Association* 267: 958–60.

Kessler, D. M., Kalk, C. E., and Singer, J. (1973). Assessing health quality—a case for tracers. *New England Journal of Medicine* 288: 189–94.

Matthews, D. A., and Feinstein, A. R. (1988). A review of systems for the personal aspects of patient care. *American Journal of Medical Sciences* 295: 159–71.

Matthews, D. A., and Feinstein, A. R. (1989). A new instrument for patients' ratings of physician performance in the hospital setting. *Journal of General Internal Medicine* 4: 14–22.

McDermott, S., and Rogers, D. E. (1983). Technology's consort. *American Journal of Medicine* 74: 353–58.

Nightingale, E. F. (1863). *Notes on Hospitals.* 3rd ed. London: Longman, Roberts & Green.

Wirth, L., ed. (1940). The quest for precision. In *Eleven Twenty-Six: A Decade of Social Science Research,* p. 169 of Roundtable Discussion: Quantification. Chicago: University of Chicago Press.

11

The Politics of Caring

ROBERT H. BINSTOCK, PH.D.

> Caring, the activity, breeds caring, the attitude, and caring, the attitude, seeds caring, the politics.
>
> D. Stone, in the *Nation*, 2000

THE PRECEDING chapters of this volume have addressed various aspects of caring needed by persons who are ill and have disabilities, as well as issues associated with the provision of caring in the United States by health care professionals, families, friends, and neighbors, and community-based voluntary organizations. This chapter explores the topic in a rather different dimension. It considers the ways in which American society *is* and *is not* a caring society with respect to the health of its people, as expressed through its national, state, and local polities—that is, through governmental actions and inactions.

Issues of health are rather similar across countries, and there are many commonalities in the ways that nations deal with them. All industrialized nations, for instance, have public health programs and license and regulate health care providers to some extent. But there are many differences among them as well, such as in their approaches to health insurance and other aspects of financing and organizing health care. Much of the variation in approaches can be traced to the histories, ideologies, and institutions of respective political systems.

The relatively unique character of the American political tradition must be at the core of any attempt to make some sense out of the patterns through which we are and are not a caring society with respect to the health of our populace. Without this context, an assessment of caring as expressed through our public sector would be ungrounded and unrealistic. Accordingly, this discussion of the politics of caring begins with a review of some of the fundamental characteristics of the American political system.

THE AMERICAN POLITICAL TRADITION

Swedish sociologist GØsta Esping-Andersen (1999) attempted to sort out the different national approaches to issues of health and social risk with a tripartite typology of the ways in which individuals view their collective responsibility for their fellow citizens. One ideal type is *Homo liberalismus,* whose ideal is to pursue his own personal welfare.

> The well-being of others is their affair, not his. A belief in noble self-reliance does not necessarily imply indifference to others. *Homo liberalismus* may be generous, even altruistic. But kindness toward others is a personal affair, not something dictated from above. His ethics tell him that a free lunch is amoral, that collectivism jeopardizes freedom, that individual liberty is a fragile good, easily sabotaged by sinister socialists or paternalistic authoritarians. *Homo liberalismus* prefers a welfare regime where those who can play the market do so, whereas those who cannot must merit charity. (171)

Another type is *Homo familius.* In sharp contrast to *Homo liberalismus:*

> he abhors atomism and impersonality and, hence, markets and individualism. His worst enemy is the Hobbesian world of elbows, because self-interest is amoral; a person will find his equilibrium when he puts himself in service of his family. Freedom, to *Homo familius,* means that he and his kin are immunized from the ceaseless threats that the greater world around him produce [*sic*]. . . . *Homo familius* wants a welfare regime that tames the market and exalts the virtues of close-knit solidarity. (171)

The third type, *Homo socialdemocraticus,* is also collectively oriented, more as a matter of cool calculation than as an act of charity.

> *Homo socialdemocraticus* plans his life around the one basic idea that he, and everybody else, will be better off in a world without want but also without free-riders. Society is something that we all are compelled to share, and so we had better share it well. . . . *Homo socialdemocraticus* is fully convinced that the more we invest in the public good, the better it will become. And this will trickle down to all, himself especially, in the

> form of a good life. Collective solutions are therefore the best single assurance of a good, if perhaps dull, individual life. (171–72)

Although all societies comprise some mixture of these types, one type or another tends to be predominant in any one nation. Esping-Andersen argues that Sweden and the United States are arguably the closest living embodiments of the dreams of, respectively, *Homo socialdemocraticus* and *Homo liberalismus.*

Liberal Ideology

Most students of American political life over the past two centuries would agree with Esping-Andersen's characterization of the United States. Indeed, in his classic and influential treatise on the American political tradition, political theorist Louis Hartz (1955) argued that our political ideas, institutions, and behavior uniquely reflect a virtually unanimous acceptance of the tenets of the English political philosopher John Locke, whose ideas were in harmony with the laissez-faire economics subsequently propounded by Adam Smith. In Hartz's view, the Lockean liberal consensus in the United States can be attributed to our nation's equally unique absence of a feudal tradition with hierarchical and paternalistic institutions. In Lockean liberalism, the individual is much more important than the collective, and one of the few important functions of a limited state is to ensure that the wealth that individuals accumulate through the market is protected. In fact, Locke (1690 [1924]) argued that governments should be dissolved if they fail to protect the rights of individuals to life, liberty, and property.

The framers of the U.S. Constitution, strongly influenced by the atomistic individualism of Locke's philosophy and his views on the sanctity of private property, took pains to limit the power of government. The constitutional rights they established for U.S. citizens are largely protections for the individual and his property from governmental actions. Americans have no constitutional rights to economic security, shelter, or health care (except for prisoners incarcerated by the state).

This ongoing ideological tradition helps to explain certain aspects of our political system's approach to issues of health. Our governments intervene a great deal in the health arena. But on some matters of health and health care we have been more inclined to rely on the free market and the voluntary sector than do most other industrialized nations. The issue of access to health care is a prime example. By and large, we have expected individuals and employers to finance personal health care. To be sure, government has intervened to finance care for specific groups of citizens that the market has failed to cover in this fashion (as is discussed in some detail below). But these interventions to redress market failures have been confined to selected "deserving" groups and have not been extended to all those whom the market leaves uninsured.

Fragmentation of Power

Even as the framers of the U.S. Constitution were enamored of Locke's political philosophy, they and many other early Americans were also heavily influenced by *The Spirit of the Laws,* written by French philosopher Baron de Montesquieu (1748 [1949]), in which he urged that the powers of governments should be separated in order to thwart the development of tyrannical states. As historian Clinton Rossiter (1953) noted, "Every literate colonist could quote [Montesquieu] to advantage, and . . . [his] exposition of the separation of powers was already making perfect sense to American minds" (359). Accordingly, the framers divided the very limited powers of the national government they established into an executive, legislative, and judicial branch—each with the power to check the actions of the other branches. This structure, of course, made it difficult for government to act and thereby interfere with the individual and his property. The importance of this arrangement for protecting the free market and property was made clear by James Madison (1787 [1937]) when he argued for the adoption of the Constitution in *The Federalist, No. 10*.

The separation of powers exacerbated what was already a characteristic of the American political system—the endemic fragmentation of power in a federal form of government. Not only did the state governments retain most of their power in the federal system but, reflecting the influence of Montesquieu, the powers in each of them were also separated. Today, the fragmentation of governmental power in the United States is astounding. Altogether, we have some eighty thousand governments: as well as the state and national governments, we have counties, municipalities, special district governments, and independent school districts—and the powers of each are usually separated and even further fragmented.

The consequence is that, in general, government intervention is very difficult in the American political system. As an elementary reminder, consider how difficult it is simply to pass legislation at the national level, whether related to health or any other matter. Majorities must be assembled among 100 senators and 435 representatives, most of them representing different constituencies. Unlike many industrial democracies, the United States lacks centralized, disciplined political parties; hence, assembling such majorities is no mean feat. The two houses of Congress then have to agree on the details of a bill and then vote again. And then the president has to agree to the legislation. In the case of health-related matters, add to the picture that most of the authority to deal with them is in the hands of the fifty separate states, their counties, their municipalities, and the special district governments that they create (e.g., the Los Angeles Air Pollution Control District)—and that, in turn, power within each of these entities is fragmented.

One consequence of this fragmentation is that even when political leaders of a *socialdemocraticus* stripe are inclined to be interventionist, the adoption and implementation of policies can be very difficult (see Binstock, Levin, and Weatherley, 1985). Consider that various American presidents in the twentieth century have failed in their efforts to secure national health insurance—most recently President Bill Clinton, who declared it the prime legislative goal of his first term (see Johnson and Broder, 1996–97). One of these presidents might well have succeeded had he been the head of a disciplined ruling party in a parliamentary system of government, with no separation of executive and legislative powers. Fragmentation of power similarly makes implementation of adopted policies difficult. For instance, although Medicaid was enacted in 1965 to ensure that selected categories of poor persons in each state would be covered by health insurance, Arizona refused to participate in the program until nearly twenty years later.

Another consequence of fragmentation is that policy interventions tend to be incremental rather than systemic or comprehensive. The difficulties of assembling legislative majorities in a system with undisciplined parties often forces political leaders to scale back their ambitious proposals and attempt to achieve their goals in a piecemeal fashion. Such was the case in 1965 when President Lyndon Johnson was thwarted in his attempt to secure national health insurance. He and his policy advisors regrouped and were able to secure the passage of Medicare, that is, national health insurance for just a single segment of the population—older persons. Their hope was that this would be the first in a series of incremental steps that would ultimately add up to universal coverage (see Ball, 1995; Cohen, 1985).

GOVERNMENT INTERVENTION IN HEALTH AND HEALTH CARE

Despite the general tendency of the American political system to rely on the market to meet the health and social needs of its citizens, and the difficulties of adopting and implementing public policies, U.S. governments actually intervene substantially in the health sector.

Health Insurance and Direct Health Care

National, state, and local governments in the United States provide health insurance and direct health care for about 100 million people. In 1999, public funds accounted for 46 percent of an estimated $1.2 trillion in national health care expenditures (Smith et al., 1999). Government tax policy also subsidizes the health insurance coverage that 67.5 million workers and their families have through employer-sponsored health plans (Fronstin, 1999). Health insurance premiums paid by employers are tax deductible as a business expense and are also excluded from workers' taxable income, as are "flexible spending accounts" that allow employees to pay for health care expenses through payroll deductions. In 1998, these subsidization policies cost the federal government $111 billion in forgone revenue (Sheils and Hogan, 1999).

The American propensity to rely on the market, however, left 16.3 percent of the U.S. population, or 44.3 million people, without health insurance coverage throughout 1998 (U.S. Census Bureau, 1999). Of twenty-nine industrialized nations that are members of the Organization for Economic Cooperation and Development (OECD), twenty-four use the power of government to assure health insurance coverage for at least 99 percent of their citizens (Anderson and Poullier, 1999). But the U.S. rate of government-assured health insurance is only 33 percent, by far the lowest. (Mexico and Turkey are the only other nations in this group that have no form of universal health insurance.)

In the context of the American political ethos, the fact that we do not use government to assure universal health insurance is neither a surprise nor a deficiency. Rather, it is a reflection of our traditional values regarding the appropriate role of government.

Nonetheless, the number of Americans without access to health care would be far higher if it were not for a series of governmental programs created to aid particular groups of citizens that have been politically legitimized as especially deserving of public help. In most instances, these expressions of societal caring have been rationalized by the fact that employer-sponsored insurance through the market does not reach them.

Among the largest of these constituencies is older Americans—about 35 million people at the beginning of the twenty-first century (Hobbs, 1996). From the mid-1930s through the mid-1970s, U.S. society constructed, in effect, an Old Age Welfare State based on compassionate stereotypes of older people as poor, frail, unable to work, socially dependent objects of discrimination, and above all, deserving (see Binstock, 1983). For more than forty years, American society accepted the oversimplified but caring notion that all older persons were essentially the same and that all were worthy of governmental assistance. The American polity implemented this compassionate construct by adopting and financing major age-categorical benefit programs—Social Security, Medicare, and many others—through which older people have been exempted from the eligibility screenings applied to welfare applicants to determine whether they are worthy of public help.

The compassionate stereotypes of older people that nourished the expansion of old-age programs eroded during the last quarter of the twentieth century as epithets such as "greedy geezers" emerged (see, e.g., Fairlie, 1988; Salholz, 1990) and policy debates frequently portrayed older people as engaged in selfish, intergenerational competition with the rest of their fellow Americans (see, e.g., Cook et al., 1994; Peterson, 1999). Nonetheless, the programs established in the era of compassionate ageism remain largely intact. Consequently, the proportion of the annual budget of the federal government devoted to benefits to older people is currently about 40 percent (Binstock, 1998a).

Medicare, on which the United States currently spends 2.5 percent of its national wealth (an estimated $220 billion in 1999) (Congressional Budget Office, 1999), provides a basic package of national health insurance to all persons aged sixty-five and older who are eligible for Social Security benefits (or Railroad Retirement Benefits)—although there are significant gaps in this coverage (discussed below). The political rationale for establishing this program in 1965 was that older people, retired from employment, had no way to obtain group health insurance. Comparatively few had employer-sponsored retiree health insurance. Most older people could not afford the comparatively steep premiums charged for individual insurance policies, and many could not obtain them because of preexisting medical conditions.

The result of this government action to establish Medicare is immedi-

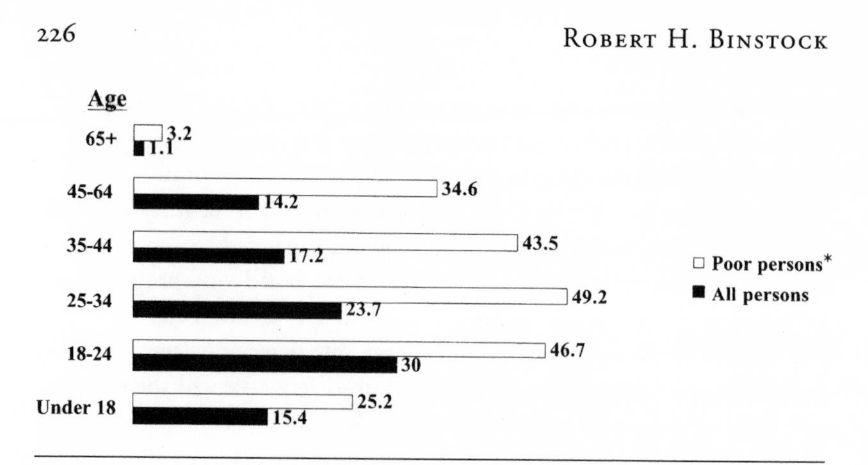

Figure 11.1. *Percentage of All Persons and Poor Persons Never Covered by Health Insurance in 1998, by Age Group*

*Income below the poverty line.
Source: U.S. Census Bureau, 1999

ately apparent in figure 11.1, which presents lack of insurance coverage by age group. Because of this program, virtually all of the 35 million Americans aged sixty-five and older have health insurance coverage, in stark contrast to people in all the other age categories. Thus, Medicare is a prime example of how access to health care can be distributed because of political decisions regarding the "deservingness" of a group.

Another selected group covered by Medicare are the 4.7 million younger people who became eligible after having received Disability Insurance (DI) benefits from the federal government for at least two years (Health Care Financing Administration, 1998). These are individuals who, due to a medically certified physical or mental impairment (but not other circumstances), are unable to engage in any kind of "substantial employment" (earning $500 monthly or more) for at least a year. They have been politically legitimized as deserving of Medicare coverage because without employment they cannot obtain group health insurance or afford it on their own. Until recently, DI recipients who were able to return to substantial employment lost their Medicare coverage after two years. However, in recognition of the fact that many employers do not provide health insurance, this disincentive to work was recently attenuated by the Ticket to Work and Work Incentives Improvement Act of 1999. This legislation enables DI recipients who become substantially employed to participate in the Medicare Program for an additional four and one-half years.

Also covered by Medicare are about 80,000 persons with end-stage renal disease. The extension of coverage to this group principally resulted from a "caring" response of a congressional committee, engendered when an advocacy group for people with this disease arranged for a patient to receive a dramatic kidney dialysis treatment while testifying at a hearing.

Some poor Americans also receive governmental support in obtaining basic health care and long-term care via the Medicaid program, a jointly funded cooperative venture between the federal and the state governments. But Medicaid policy does not fully equate poverty with "deservingness." Federal law requires only that states provide coverage for specific categories of deserving groups among the poor that, in their nature, are unlikely to be able to obtain employer-sponsored insurance through the market. Although the list of these required categories is long and detailed (see Health Care Financing Administration, 1998), the principal eligible groups are children, adults with dependent children, disabled persons (who are not eligible for federal DI benefits), blind persons, and older people (to cover their long-term care expenses, not covered by Medicare, as well as their Medicare Part A Hospital Insurance deductibles and copayments, and their premiums for Part B Supplementary Medical Insurance). Persons within these categories are eligible for Medicaid if their income and financial assets fall below thresholds determined by each state (within minimum federal guidelines). States also have the option of providing Medicaid coverage for other categories, including the "medically needy." Altogether, Medicaid covered 40.6 million persons in 1997 (Kaiser Commission, 1999). Of these, 52 percent were children, 21 percent were adults in families with dependent children (the vast majority of whom were women), 17 percent were blind or disabled, and 10 percent were older people. However, 72 percent of all Medicaid spending was on behalf of the elderly and disabled, primarily because of the large costs of long-term care. Combined federal and state Medicaid expenditures for 1999 were estimated at $188 billion.

The responsiveness of American society to these deserving groups varies throughout the nation because states can be more and less generous in establishing income and asset thresholds, as well as in how readily they enable people who are potentially eligible to be covered by Medicaid. Consider, for example, the range of low-income thresholds used by states to determine whether infants are eligible for Medicaid (Ellwood and Lewis, 1999). At the most generous end of the continuum, Tennessee's threshold is 400 percent of the federal poverty line, Rhode Island's is 250 percent, and in California, Maryland, and Massachusetts it is 200 percent.

At the other extreme is a threshold of 133 percent, employed by Alabama, Alaska, Colorado, Louisiana, Montana, North Dakota, Oregon, South Dakota, Utah, Virginia, and Wyoming (Ku, Ullman, and Almeida, 1999). (For poor persons who do not qualify for Medicaid through the eligible-population categories, most states have established a general medical assistance program. Such programs are supported by state funds only; they tend to be less generous in their financial eligibility thresholds and coverage than is Medicaid.)

Congress underscored the federal government's commitment to poor children as a specially deserving group in 1997 when it established a new Children's Health Insurance Program (CHIP). In addition to allowing states to redesign or expand their existing Medicaid programs, CHIP provided $24 billion to the states (over five years) to expand Medicaid eligibility and other forms of health insurance coverage for an estimated 3.1 million children who were not otherwise insured. Again, states have varied in the generosity of the poverty thresholds they have established for this program; for example, Vermont's is 300 percent of the poverty line; Arizona's is 150 percent (Ku, Ullman, and Almeida, 1999). In addition, the outreach efforts of states have been markedly different. During the first six months of 1999, for example, California, Florida, Georgia, and New York made substantial progress; Texas made no progress; and Wyoming and Washington had not even submitted plans to participate in the program (Smith, 1999).

Two additional groups—veterans and Native Americans—have been singled out for government assistance with health care, but for reasons other than market failure. The political legitimacy of veterans as beneficiaries of government support arises, of course, from their military service on behalf of the nation. This legitimacy has been substantially reinforced since the Civil War (see Skocpol, 1992) by a well-organized and politically influential veterans lobby. Government provision of health care for veterans in the United States dates from the Revolutionary War. Then, and through the early twentieth century, direct medical and hospital care was primarily provided by state and local governments (U.S. Department of Veterans Affairs, 1999). Although the first domiciliary and medical facility for veterans was authorized by the federal government in 1811, the modern Veterans Administration (VA) health care system, funded and operated by the national government, was not established until 1930 (Wetle and Rowe, 1984). The VA system operates within a fixed budget, about $17 billion in 1999. Although all veterans (presently, about 25 million) are technically eligible for VA health care, the system stays within its budget by establishing priority groups for care eligibility. The highest priority is for veterans with "service-connected conditions resulting in disability of 50 percent or more" (U.S. General Accounting Office, 1999a).

The federal government directly provides health care to Native Americans pursuant to its "trust responsibility" arising from treaties executed between 1784 and the late 1800s. The Indian Health Service, with a budget of $2.2 billion, operates a comprehensive health service delivery system for about 1.5 million "American Indians" and "Alaska Natives" (Indian Health Service, 1999).

Other Forms of Governmental Intervention

In addition to these efforts for groups that have been politically legitimized as deserving, the federal, state, and local governments also provide health insurance benefits, as well as direct health care, for their own employees. For instance, the U.S. Department of Defense operates a health care system, funded at $15.6 billion in 1999, for which some 8.2 million active military personnel, their dependents, and military retirees and their dependents are eligible for care (U.S. General Accounting Office, 1999b).

However, the range of activities by which government enhances the availability and quality of health care and improves and protects health status extends far beyond providing health insurance and direct care. Government activity includes public health programs, training for health care professionals, health-related research, and a substantial amount of regulation of private-sector health insurance companies and health care operations.

Public Health Efforts. The public health system in the United States is reputed to be the most advanced in the world. It is safe to say that it has far more impact in enhancing the health of Americans than medical care for individuals. As Surgeon General David Satcher observed in 1999, "Americans enjoy better health conditions and live longer than at any time in the past. To a large extent these trends are the result of the tremendous efforts of public health" (quoted in Trafford, 1999).

The states, counties, and most large municipalities have public health departments that are responsible for promoting health and quality of life by preventing and controlling disease, injury, and disability. The national focal point for such efforts is the federal government's Centers for Disease Control and Prevention (CDC), which in 1999, for example, had an annual budget of $2.9 billion (Centers for Disease Control and Prevention, 1999). The range of public health activities in which CDC engages is extensive, including programs in chronic disease prevention and health promotion, environmental health, food safety, genetics and disease prevention, immunization, infectious diseases, injury prevention and control, occupational safety and health, and epidemiological surveillance that is global in scope.

Training for Health-Care Professionals. The federal government plays a major role in the financing of graduate medical education (i.e., post–medical school) for physicians. Its primary means of doing this has been through payments from the Medicare program for residency training in more than twelve hundred teaching hospitals throughout the country. In 1997, Medicare paid almost $7 billion for graduate medical education, about two-thirds of it for indirect costs (Medicare Payment Advisory Commission, 1998).

In addition, comparatively minor programs for health care training are carried out by other agencies. The National Health Service Corps provides scholarships and loans as a means of recruiting health care professionals who subsequently provide services to the "medically underserved" (Mullan, 1999). Part of the mission of the Health Resources and Services Administration is to improve the workforce capacity and practices of health professions, particularly in primary medical care and public health, through educational programs (Health Resources and Services Administration, 1999).

Research. The federal government also plays a leading role in funding research that acquires new knowledge to help prevent, detect, diagnose, and treat disease and disability. The principal vehicle for this role is the National Institutes of Health (NIH), comprising twenty-five institutes and centers, some of which (e.g., the National Cancer Institute) are focused on diseases. NIH currently spends nearly $16 billion a year (National Institutes of Health, 1999) to fund research in its own laboratories; support the research of nonfederal scientists in universities, medical schools, and hospitals; finance the training of research investigators; and foster communication of biomedical and health care information.

A number of other federal agencies also conduct and sponsor health-related research and training. In addition to its public health programs, the CDC operates a Center for Health Statistics. The Agency for Healthcare Research and Quality funds both intramural and extramural health services research focused on measuring and improving the quality of health care, reducing its costs, broadening access to services, and translating evidence-based research into clinical practice and into practical information for consumers and other health care purchasers. Many other components of the U.S. Department of Health and Human Services also carry out health-related research. Among them are the Health Care Financing Administration (which administers the Medicare and Medicaid programs), the Administration on Aging, the Administration for Children and Families, the Substance Abuse and Mental Health Services Administration, and the Office of the Assistant Secretary for Planning and Evaluation.

Regulation. Even as government has done a great deal to nurture the nation's health through these various programs, it has been very active in regulating the private health care sector. Most hospitals, nursing homes, home health agencies, hospices, and other health care provider organizations are subject to a plethora of regulations regarding safety and quality of patient care. Prior to the enactment of Medicare and Medicaid in 1965, such regulations were primarily established and enforced by the states pursuant to their general responsibilities for basic health and welfare. Since then, because most health care organizations participate in the Medicare and Medicaid programs, they have become increasingly subject to federal regulations. Some of these have been enacted to compensate for perceived inadequacies in state regulation, such as measures to reform the quality of nursing home care established in the Omnibus Budget Reconciliation Act of 1987. Others have responded to new developments in thinking about appropriate patient care. For instance, in the context of growing ethical concerns about patient autonomy, the federal Patient Self-Determination Act was enacted in 1990, requiring health care organizations immediately to inform new patients of their rights to refuse medical and surgical treatment and to execute written legal documents, "advance directives," regarding their preferences in this regard.

The licensing of health care professionals and regulation of private health insurance plans has also traditionally been the bailiwick of state governments. In recent years, however, the federal government has become very active in the insurance arena. For instance, in 1996 alone, it enacted three laws imposing requirements on the insurance industry, each intended to benefit consumers directly. The Mental Health Parity Act of 1996 responded to the entreaties of mental health advocates by requiring that if a group insurance plan covers mental health, the annual and lifetime benefits available must be equivalent to those available for medical and surgical services. The

Newborns' and Mothers' Health Protection Act of 1996, enacted in response to numerous anecdotal reports of "drive by" births, mandated minimum inpatient stays for mothers and their newborns following deliveries and cesarean sections. And the Health Insurance Portability and Accountability Act of 1996 made obtaining group health insurance easier for individuals with preexisting health problems and disabilities or previous illnesses and for those who have lost their coverage because of changing jobs or job termination.

In addition, health insurers and health care providers are subject to implicit "yardstick regulation" by the decisions that the federal Health Care Financing Administration (HCFA) and state governments make regarding the services that Medicare and Medicaid will cover, and the prices they will pay for them. For example, as expensive new surgical and diagnostic procedures (such as organ transplants and magnetic resonance imaging) are developed, private insurers are typically slow to cover them, designating them as only "experimental." However, if HCFA decides to cover them for its nearly 40 million Medicare enrollees, the insurance industry feels pressure to "measure up" to the model established by government. In those circumstances, it becomes very difficult for the industry to maintain the posture that such procedures and tests are experimental. By the same token, Medicare payment policies can implicitly regulate the fees that health care providers charge private payers. In the early 1980s, for instance, Medicare implemented a policy of reimbursing hospitals for inpatients with flat fees, based on a patient's primary diagnosis. This, in turn, enabled insurance companies to place effective pressure on hospitals to reduce their "private-pay" charges to better conform to the Medicare rates.

One further important area of government regulation in the health arena is the consumer protection activities of the federal Food and Drug Administration (FDA). This agency is responsible for ensuring that medicines, medical devices, blood supplies, and certain experimental medical treatments (e.g., gene therapy) are safe and effective, and that foods and cosmetics are truthfully labeled and not harmful. The FDA (with a budget in 1999 of about $1 billion) regulates more than $1 trillion worth of products annually (Food and Drug Administration, 1999).

A TRAJECTORY OF CARING

It can be seen from the preceding overview that the extent of governmental activity in the health arena is quite remarkable, given that it has developed within a nation that has a political tradition characterized by Lockean liberalism and substantial fragmentation of public sector power. Through incremental steps over many years, governmental intervention on behalf of the health of Americans has become extensive. This trajectory of governmental caring is likely to continue.

One very general reason that government intervention in the health arena is likely to increase is the contrast between what our country spends on health care and what our people feel about our health care system. The United States devotes far more of its private and public resources to health care than do the other industrialized nations of the world. This country spends 13.5 percent of its gross domestic product (GDP) on health care, compared with a median of 7.5 percent for the twenty-nine OECD nations (Anderson and Poullier, 1999). And U.S. per capita spending on health care is $3,925, compared with the OECD median of $1,728. (A far-distant second to the United States is Switzerland, where per capita spending is $2,547.) Yet Americans in the aggregate are not at all content with what this comparative plenitude of resources produces. In a recent survey of satisfaction with health care systems in five nations—Australia, Canada, New Zealand, the United Kingdom, and the United States—nearly half of the American public (46%) felt that "there are some good things in our health system, but fundamental changes are needed to make it work" (Donelan et al., 1999: 208). An additional 33 percent of Americans expressed a considerably more negative view, saying that "our health care system has so much wrong with it that we need to completely rebuild it" (208). (In contrast, even though per capita spending on health care in the United Kingdom is only about one-third of what it is in the United States, only 14 percent of people in that nation felt that a complete rebuilding was needed.) This general dissatisfaction will probably manifest itself in terms of movements for specific reforms as our health care system continues to undergo rapid changes. A contemporary example is governmental responses to the ascendance of managed care, such as the enactment of patients' rights bills in many states, and additional legislation on this matter that is pending in Congress.

We can also anticipate increased governmental intervention for two other reasons. One reason is that there are a number of specific forces in contemporary society that will continuously bring new health-related issues to the fore. The other is that there are long-standing unresolved issues susceptible to government action that remain more or less active on the policy agenda, such as whether and how to insure the uninsured.

Forces Generating New Issues

In his study of democracy in America in the first half of the nineteenth century, the Frenchman Alexis de Tocqueville was particularly struck by the omnipresence and influence of voluntary associations in the United States.

> Americans of all ages, all conditions, and all dispositions constantly form associations. . . . The Americans make associations to give entertainments, to found seminaries, to build inns, to construct churches, to diffuse books, to send missionaries to the antipodes; in this manner they found hospitals, prisons, and schools. . . . Wherever at the head of some new undertaking you see the government in France, or a man of rank in England, in the United States you will be sure to find an association. (de Tocqueville, 1945: 114)

In recent decades, voluntary associations (read as advocacy and interest groups) have become a major force in the generation of new health-related issues for the public agenda. They also work continually, and often effectively, to achieve their policy goals. In the early 1970s, for example, the Gerontological Society of America (GSA), comprising biologists, physicians, and other professionals who are focused on issues of aging, played the lead role in proposing and securing the establishment of a National Institute on Aging (NIA) (Lockett, 1983). Subsequent continual lobbying by the Alzheimer's Association helped an earmarked NIA appropriation for Alzheimer disease research to grow from $800,000 in 1976 to $350 million in 1998: then, the association set a goal of securing a $500 million earmarked budget in 2001 (Binstock, 1998b).

Today, more than a hundred national voluntary health associations (VHAS) and coalitions among them push forward a public policy agenda in the health arena to benefit their respective constituencies. Although many VHAS began with the mission of direct service to patients and their families, as well as raising funds for biomedical research, within the past twenty-five years they have come to understand that systemwide changes accomplished through public policy provide enormous leverage. The president and CEO of the Arthritis Foundation, for example, has stated, "We can more quickly achieve our mission for the individual with arthritis by leveraging our limited resources to achieve a greater impact on the population as a whole through affecting the policies and systems of government and the health care delivery process" (Riggins, 1998: 40).

Most VHAS have established public policy offices in the Washington,

D.C., metropolitan area so that they can readily participate in the policy process on a daily basis (Binstock, 1998b). Some also have state and regional policy offices. The larger VHAS devote substantial annual budgets to their policy activities (e.g., the American Cancer Society, $6.2 million; the American Heart Association, $1.5 million).

The importance of the role that voluntary health associations play in public policy and the political legitimacy that they have attained were officially institutionalized in 1999. In response to a report issued by the Institute of Medicine (1998), the National Institutes of Health has established a Director's Council of Public Representatives to facilitate interaction between NIH and the general public in setting NIH research priorities. In keeping with explicit recommendations from the Institute of Medicine, the director's appointments to the council specifically included representatives from "disease specific interest groups" and "advocates for patients or special populations."

The majority of VHA national lobbying efforts are directed toward members of Congress and their staffs, although substantial attention is focused on federal administrative and regulatory agencies. They mobilize their constituencies for advocacy purposes through public policy modules developed on internet web sites and using listservs, "blast" faxes, automatic mailgrams and telegrams, voicemail, and telephone "patch-throughs" to congressional offices. Some of them have also developed computerized databases that match grassroots advocates with congressional districts and key congressional contacts, and they track those individuals within their constituencies who have previously responded to VHA "action alerts."

VHAS and VHA coalitions advocate for an extraordinary range of public interventions. Broadly speaking, they seek increased funding for biomedical, epidemiological, and health services research; expanded governmental service and public health programs; favorable decisions in the regulation of food and drugs and approval of new therapeutic regimes; regulations and programs that support people with disabilities in everyday life; patients' rights in health care settings and in the processes of obtaining insurance; and government intervention to improve health care quality and access, including expanded insurance coverage for specific medical treatments and tests, and for uninsured persons. In the aggregate, VHAS pursue innumerable specific goals within each of these areas.

The policy agendas of VHAS and other advocates in the health arena are continually fueled with new issues by other forces in contemporary society. Our capacities to monitor health status and health care quality increasingly become more sophisticated. A burgeoning industry of biological research, randomized trials, and epidemiological studies constantly improves our understanding of factors that affect health and health care outcomes, with implications for possible public interventions. In addition, technological and biomedical discoveries and innovations generate questions of fairness and equity that lend themselves to the possibility of government intervention, such as whether genetic testing should be allowed to be used as a screen to exclude applicants for private insurance or how societal scarce resources (e.g., transplant organs) should be distributed.

Ongoing Issues

The agenda for government action with respect to health grows ever larger because the new issues that constantly arise hardly obliterate ongoing issues that flow from previous public interventions and policy proposals. Some of these ongoing matters involve the need to achieve better implementation of existing policies—for example, the Children's Health Insurance Program (see Pear, 2000a). Others involve efforts to deepen and broaden the nature of government's intervention in areas where it is already involved, but only a little bit to date. An example of this is family caregiving, an issue dealt with in minimal fashion by the Family Medical Leave Act of 1993, which mandated noncompensated leave of up to twelve weeks for employees of large firms, but only for employees who have worked at least 1,250 hours during the preceding twelve months and who are caring for immediate family members (i.e., not for extended family). Advocates are now pressing to strengthen this legislation to make it require that caregivers be paid during their leave, increase the number of covered employers, and broaden the definition of whom can be cared for by the worker on leave (see Hudson and Gonyea, 2000).

Still other issues concern areas in which, although government is already heavily involved, there are important gaps in present policy. Currently, the most politically prominent of these areas is the health care of older people. Although older Americans have had national health insurance since 1965, they have important health needs that are not covered: outpatient prescription drugs; routine physical exams, eye exams, and dental services; eyeglasses and hearing aids; and extended hospital stays. For some of these needs, the federal government seems poised to continue its trajectory of caring. Coverage for prescription drugs—essential for treatment of chronic illnesses that are highly prevalent among older people—in mid-2000 appeared to be the most likely of these gaps to be covered in the near term (see Pear, 2000b). Although Medicare home health services and Medicaid have provided long-term care coverage for some older persons, financing such care is a major burden for many elderly and their families (see Binstock and Cluff, 2000). Policy proposals for expanded public financing of long-term care have repeatedly surfaced since the late 1980s, including a relatively minor initiative set forth by President Clinton in 2000 (White House press release, 2000). A significant new program of government-financed long-term care is likely to be established when many members of the baby-boom cohort reach old age, if not sooner, because of the greatly increasing number of persons in need of such care. And also, because of the aging of the baby boomers, the nation will need to greatly increase its financial commitment to Medicare if the program is to be sustained (see Vladeck, 1999a). The proportion of national wealth (i.e., GDP) spent on Medicare in 1998 was 2.5 percent; it is projected to more than double, to 5.3 percent, in 2025, when most baby boomers will be aged at least sixty-five (Moon, 1999).

One matter on which it is not at all clear that the trajectory of caring will proceed is government action to assure that all Americans have health insurance. As noted at the outset of this chapter, 16.3 percent of the U.S. population had no health insurance coverage throughout 1998 (U.S. Census Bureau, 1999). The percentage without insurance was about double that (32.3%) among the poor; that is, people with incomes below the federal poverty line. (The poverty line varies in relation to the size and composition of a household; for instance, in 1998 it was $13,120 for a household of three that included one child, $16,530 for a household of four, with two children [Dalaker, 1999].) Race and ethnicity also clearly have a strong bearing on whether or not people have health insurance (see figure 11.2). Blacks and Asian and Pacific Islanders are about twice as likely to be uninsured as non-Hispanic whites; persons of Hispanic origin are about three times as likely to be uninsured. However, poverty status tends to level the groupings; for instance, the percentage of poor, non-Hispanic whites who have no insurance is about the same as for poor blacks.

Although employer-sponsored health plans are a major source of insurance, being employed is hardly a guarantee of coverage. Only slightly more than half of all workers (53.3%) have employment-sponsored health insurance (U.S. Census Bureau, 1999). The percentage of covered workers varies substantially in relation to the size of the employer's firm. Only 29.3 percent of workers in firms with fewer than twenty-five employees have

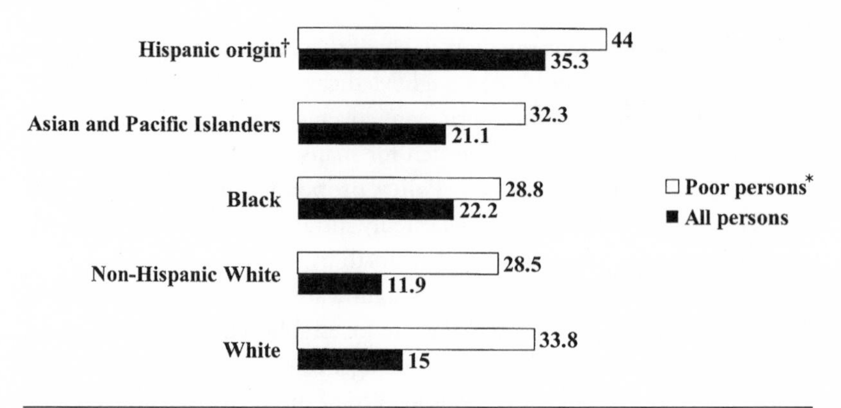

Figure 11.2. *Percentage of All Persons and Poor Persons Never Covered by Health Insurance in 1998, by Race and Ethnicity*

*Income below the poverty line.
†Persons of Hispanic origin may be of any race.
Source: U.S. Census Bureau, 1999

insurance, while two-thirds of workers are covered in firms that employ five hundred workers or more. As shown in figure 11.3, nearly one-fifth of people who worked during 1998 were never insured. To be sure, people who worked full-time were more likely to have coverage than part-timers. However, nearly one-half of the poor people who worked—full-time as well as part-time—were uninsured. Ironically, their rate of coverage was worse than for those poor persons who did not work at all. This is because government insurance programs cover large numbers of nonworking poor persons.

Current trends in the labor market suggest that, for the foreseeable future, the outlook for expansion of health insurance coverage through the private sector is dim. Although the percentage of employed Americans has grown to its highest level in many decades, during the economic expansion that began in the 1990s, employer-sponsored health care benefits have not grown commensurably. In the absence of a new government health insurance initiative that reaches beyond the present selection of politically legitimated groups, it is unlikely that many of the 44 million uninsured Americans will be covered; indeed, the number of uninsured may grow.

From the 1920s through the early 1990s, various presidents have attempted, unsuccessfully, to establish some form of universal coverage.

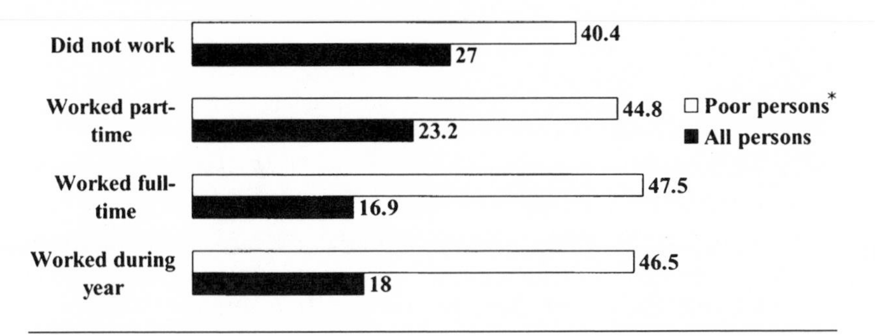

Figure 11.3. *Percentage of All Persons and Poor Persons Never Covered by Health Insurance in 1998, by Employment Status*

*Income below the poverty line.
Source: U.S. Census Bureau, 1999

When and how might such an effort be renewed and have a chance of success?

The proportion of voters who are poor and members of racial and ethnic minority groups will grow sharply over the next several decades. And if current trends in employee health insurance continue, the proportions of uninsured Americans in these categories will probably increase. Perhaps they will be mobilized effectively to demand access to the health care that their fellow citizens receive.

A far likelier scenario is that the swiftly changing dynamics of American health care will threaten profits in the health care industry. Government insurance for an additional 44 million people (and perhaps a larger number in the future) would be a bountiful source of revenue. Unlike the American Medical Association, which vigorously opposed President Johnson's attempt to secure universal insurance in 1965, today's health care industry might appreciate what can be done for it by government. As a former administrator of the federal Health Care Financing Administration has noted, Medicare financing has largely built and sustained the modern medical industrial complex (Vladeck, 1999b). The political power of the health care industry is substantial and might very well carry the day for universal coverage if united by a vision of what further governmental largesse could do for it. If so, despite a political tradition that has been dominated by a *Homo liberalismus* ethos, the United States will take its place in the first rank of caring polities, at least with respect to the health of its citizens.

REFERENCES

Anderson, G. F., and Poullier, J.-P. (1999). Health spending, access, and outcomes: Trends in industrialized countries. *Health Affairs* 18(3): 178–92.

Ball, R. M. (1995). What Medicare's architects had in mind. *Health Affairs* 14(4): 62–72.

Binstock, R. H. (1983). The aged as scapegoat. *Gerontologist* 23: 136–43.

Binstock, R. H. (1998a). Public policies on aging in the twenty-first century. *Stanford Law and Policy Review* 9(2): 311–28.

Binstock, R. H. (1998b). *Public Policy and Voluntary Health Agencies.* Washington, DC: National Health Council.

Binstock, R. H., and Cluff, L. E. (2000). Issues and challenges in home care. In R. H. Binstock and L. E. Cluff, eds., *Home Care Advances: Essential Research and Policy Issues,* pp. 3–34. New York: Springer Publishing.

Binstock, R. H., Levin, M. A., and Weatherley, R. (1985). Political dilemmas of social intervention. In R. H. Binstock and E. Shanas, eds., *Handbook of Aging and the Social Sciences,* 2nd ed., pp. 589–618. New York: Van Nostrand Reinhold.

Centers for Disease Control and Prevention (1999). About CDC. Downloaded September 3: www.cdc.gov.

Cohen, W. J. (1985). Reflections on the enactment of Medicare and Medicaid. *Health Care Financing Review,* annual supplement: 3–11.

Congressional Budget Office (1999). *The Economic and Budget Outlook: Fiscal Years 2000–2009.* Washington, DC: U.S. Government Printing Office.

Cook, F. L., Marshall, V. W., Marshall, J. G., and Kaufman, J. E. (1994). The salience of intergenerational equity in Canada and the United States. In T. R. Marmor, T. M. Smeeding, and V. L. Greene, eds., *Economic Security and Intergenerational Justice: A Look at North America,* pp. 91–129. Washington, DC: Urban Institute Press.

Dalaker, J. (1999). *Poverty in the United States: 1998.* U.S. Census Bureau, Current Population Reports, series P60-207. Washington, DC: U.S. Government Printing Office.

de Tocqueville, A. (1945). *Democracy in America,* vol. 2. New York: Vintage Books.

Donelan, K., Blendon, R. J., Schoen, C., Davis, K., and Binns, K. (1999). The cost of health system change: Public discontent in five nations. *Health Affairs* 18(3): 206–16.

Ellwood, M. R., and Lewis, K. (1999). *On and Off Medicaid: Enrollment Patterns for California and Florida in 1995.* Washington, DC: Urban Institute Press.

Esping-Andersen, G. (1999). *Social Foundations of Postindustrial Economics.* New York: Oxford University Press.

Fairlie, H. (1988). Talkin' 'bout my generation. *New Republic* 198(13): 19–22.

Food and Drug Administration (1999). The Food and Drug Administration: An overview. Downloaded September 3: www.fda.gov.

Fronstin, P. (1999). *Employment-Based Health Benefits: Who Is Offered Coverage vs.*

Who Takes It. EBRI issue brief no. 213. Washington, DC: Employee Benefit Research Institute.

Hartz, L. (1955). *The Liberal Tradition in America.* New York: Harcourt, Brace.

Health Care Financing Administration (1998). Medicare and Medicaid statistical supplement, 1998. Health Care Financing Review.

Health Resources and Services Administration (1999). Overview of programs. Downloaded September 3: www.hrsa.gov.

Hobbs, F. B. (1996). *65+ in the United States.* U.S. Bureau of the Census, Current Population Reports, special studies, P23-190. Washington, DC: U.S. Government Printing Office.

Hudson, R. B., and Gonyea, J. G. (2000). Time not yet money: The politics and promise of the Family Medical Leave Act. *Journal of Aging and Social Policy* 11 (2–3): 189–200.

Indian Health Service (1999). Fact sheet. Downloaded September 3: www.ihs.gov.

Institute of Medicine, Committee on the NIH Research Priority-Setting Process (1998). *Scientific Opportunities and Public Needs: Improving Priority-Setting and Public Input at the National Institutes of Health.* Washington, DC: National Academy Press.

Johnson, S., and Broder, D. S. (1996–97). *The System: The American Way of Politics at the Breaking Point.* Boston, MA: Little, Brown.

Kaiser Commission on Medicaid and the Uninsured (1999). *Medicaid: A Primer.* Washington, DC: Kaiser.

Ku, L., Ullman, F., and Almeida, R. (1999). *What Counts? Determining Medicaid and CHIP Eligibility for Children.* Washington, DC: Urban Institute Press.

Locke, J. (1690 [1924]). *Of Civil Government: Two Treatises.* London: Dent.

Lockett, B. A. (1983). *Aging, Politics, and Research: Setting the Federal Agenda for Research on Aging.* New York: Springer Publishing.

Madison, J. (1787 [1937]). The Federalist No. 10. In A. Hamilton, J. Jay, and J. Madison, *The Federalist: A Commentary on the Constitution of the United States,* pp. 53–62. Reprint, New York: Random House.

Medicare Payment Advisory Commission (MPAC) (1998). *Health Care Spending and the Medicare Program: A Data Book.* Washington, DC: MPAC.

Montesquieu, B. de (1748 [1949]). *The Spirit of the Laws.* Trans. T. Nugent. Reprint, New York: Hafner.

Moon, M. (1999). *Growth in Medicare Spending: What Will Beneficiaries Pay?* New York: Commonwealth Fund.

Mullan, F. (1999). The muscular samaritan: The National Health Service Corps in the new century. *Health Affairs* 18(2): 168–75.

National Institutes of Health (1999). General background information—National Institutes of Health (NIH). Downloaded September 3: www.nih.gov.

Pear, R. (2000a). Clinton to broaden effort in children's health coverage. *New York Times,* January 11, p. A14.

Pear, R. (2000b). Senate chairman offers proposal on drug benefits. *New York Times,* July 12, p. A1.

Peterson, P. G. (1999). *Gray Dawn: How the Coming Age Wave Will Transform America—and the World.* New York: Times Books.

Riggins, D. (1998). Facsimile message to the author, November 25.

Rossiter, C. (1953). *Seedtime of the Republic.* New York: Harcourt, Brace, & World.

Salholz, E. (1990). Blaming the voters: Hapless budgeteers single out "greedy geezers." *Newsweek,* October 29, p. 36.

Sheils, J., and Hogan, P. (1999). Cost of tax-exempt health benefits in 1998. *Health Affairs* 18(2): 176–81.

Skocpol, T. (1992). *Protecting Soldiers and Mothers: The Political Origins of Social Policy in the United States.* Cambridge: Harvard University Press (Belknap).

Smith, S., Heffler, S., Freeland, M., and the National Health Expenditures Projection Team (1999). The next decade of health spending: A new outlook. *Health Affairs* 18(3): 86–95.

Smith, V. K. (1999). *Enrollment Increases in State CHIP Programs: December 1998 to June 1999.* Report prepared for the Kaiser Commission on Medicaid and the Uninsured. Washington, DC: Health Management Associates.

Stone, D. (2000). Why we need a care movement. *Nation* 270(10): 13–15.

Trafford, A. (1999). A century of change. *Washington Post,* April 6, p. Z6.

U.S. Census Bureau (1999). *Health Insurance Coverage: 1998.* Current Population Survey, P60-208, October.

U.S. Department of Veterans Affairs (1999). Department of Veterans Affairs (VA): A brief history. DVA history factsheet. Downloaded August 30: www.va.gov.

U.S. General Accounting Office (1999a). *VA Health Care: Progress and Challenges in Providing Care to Veterans.* Washington, DC: U.S. Government Printing Office.

U.S. General Accounting Office (1999b). *Defense Health Care: Claims Processing Improvements Are Underway but Further Enhancements Are Needed.* Washington, DC: U.S. Government Printing Office.

Vladeck, B. C. (1999a). Plenty of nothing—a report from the Medicare commission. *New England Journal of Medicine* 340: 1503–6.

Vladeck, B. C. (1999b). The political economy of Medicare: Medicare reform requires political reform. *Health Affairs* 18(1): 22–36.

Wetle, T., and Rowe, J. W., eds. (1984). *Older Veterans: Linking VA and Community Resources.* Cambridge: Harvard University Press.

White House, The (2000). The President triples his long-term care tax credit and urges Congress to pass a long-term care initiative in 2000. Press Secretary, January 19: www.pub.whitehouse.gov/uri-r . . . //oma.eop.gov.uss.

SUMMARY

THE NEED for caring has always been part of the human condition. Whether provided by families, friends, communities, or health professionals, caring helps us to bear pain, suffering, and disability and to restore our physical, psychological, and social functioning. Moreover, as Daniel Callahan observes, even if we can bear pain and suffering and can function in our daily lives, the presence, concern, and empathy of others can provide us with the moral and psychological strength for our otherwise private struggles. When we need caring, some dimensions of what we require are common for most of us, regardless of our particular conditions. Yet, as Callahan also points out, effective caring requires attention to what each individual needs in terms of his or her particular circumstances, at that particular time, and in that particular family or social situation.

Most of us need caring to help us cope with illnesses and disabilities at some time during our lives. The nature and sources of caring may vary substantially, of course, in relation to the particular health conditions we are experiencing, our stage in the life course, and our familial, social, and economic situations. For some of us, the need for caring is intermittent, occasioned by episodes of acute illness, injury, or other trauma. But for those of us who have serious chronic illnesses and disabilities, caring is needed over extended periods of time, often many years, so that we can carry out functions that are essential to daily life. Although there are commonalities in the extended caring needed by people with severe chronic illnesses and disabilities, A. E. Benjamin and Leighton Cluff draw attention to the rather diverse needs of children with special health needs, adults with developmental disabilities, adults with physical disabilities, adults with chronic mental illness, and older adults with chronic conditions. Burton Reifler and Nancy Cox amplify this point with an extended treatment of what they term the "endless caring" that families provide to young, middle-aged, and older adults who have severe and persistent mental illness. They also make clear that these caring family members are, themselves, in need of caring.

The elements of caring—such as compassion, listening, empathy, counseling, support, and giving of time and oneself—are most readily available from the members of one's immediate family and close friends. Yet, in earlier eras, such as the American colonial period, caring was a communal obligation as well, especially among members of religious communities. In the nineteenth century and well into the twentieth century, physicians also played a major role in caring. As Joel Howell argues, there were fewer social boundaries between the profession of medicine and the ordinary citizen then; physicians were more inclined than now to regard caring as part of their mission, much like the clergy. Moreover, nineteenth-century medical theories tended to promote caring because, Howell notes, sickness was not so much ascribed to a specific disease as regarded as a condition affecting the entire human organism. Each person and temperament was unique, and therapy needed to be individualized. Getting to know the patient well was an essential part of medical practice. The rise of allopathic medicine in the late nineteenth and early twentieth centuries, with its emphasis on the natural sciences, standardization of laboratory observations, and delineation of diseases, began to reshape the role of the physician. As Howell puts it, the physician was increasingly drawn away from the bedside and into the laboratory and the surgical amphitheater. Concomitantly, the growth of professional nursing increasingly led to nurses taking over some of the caring roles of physicians. And the rise of the modern hospital and the nursing home took some of the caring function away from the family and the community.

Today, Eric Cassell asserts, caring is simply defined as outside the realm of mainstream medicine. Medical thinking is ruled by the worldview of contemporary biological science, which values atomistic, verifiable facts and undervalues the moral. Objectivity ranks much higher than subjectivity. These perspectives have created a subject/object duality that further separates humans from their own bodies. The growth and development of the bioethics movement in the second half of the twentieth century has also contributed to the erosion of caring in medical care. Born in the 1960s, a period in which the social ideal of commonality in American values gave way to pride in diversity, modern bioethics emphasizes that the autonomy of the patient should take precedence over the benevolence of the physician. It has thereby diminished and rendered nostalgic the importance and centrality of the relationship, the moral bond, between patient and physician. Moreover, Cassell argues, the grip of reductive and oversimplifying technology on medical practice and physician behavior is so strong that it has squeezed out the personal and diagnostic skills of the physician. In addition, contemporary patterns in the organization and financing of health care create disincentives for physicians to engage in caring.

What can be done to restore caring as a central concern of ordinary medical practice, not just among those physicians who are especially compassionate? Cassell calls for a redress of what he sees as the exclusivity of biological science in medical education through the development of curricular materials to teach caring, although he acknowledges that the problem of changing the nature of medical education is daunting. As an alternative, he suggests that the early days of the hospice movement be emulated through a small group of training programs focused on restoring the importance of caring, which could generate a cohesive community of adherents separate from the mainstream of medicine.

Kenneth Ludmerer and Renée Fox emphasize that the fundamental prerequisite for physicians to be caring is for them to have sufficient time with their patients. Yet, as they document, in today's economically driven health care environment, time, in the name of efficiency, is being squeezed out of patient care. Consequently, changes in the medical curriculum may not be sufficient to restore caring as integral to the practice of medicine as undertaken by new cohorts of physicians. A significant part of the teaching and learning of caring takes place implicitly, in ways that are not didactically a part of the curriculum and that are not always intended or recognized by educators, through the internal culture of the academic health center. This culture includes the modes of medical practice undertaken by clinical faculty who serve as role models and mentors. They are susceptible to the same commercial atmosphere as other contemporary physicians, in which the good visit is the short visit, patients are "consumers," and administrators speak more often of the balance sheet than of service and the relief of suffering. Clinical faculty have little time to convey what caring is about. Ludmerer and Fox believe that medical students and house officers will be able to learn about and practice caring medicine only if medical leaders have the courage to restore the internal culture of academic health centers so that they are once again less commercial and more caring. These leaders must be willing to stand up for the interests of patients and the public.

Caring has traditionally been integral to nursing practice. In hospitals, nursing homes, outpatient settings, and home care and hospice programs, nurses administer medicines; change dressings; assess patients' physical, emotional, and social states; teach patients to carry out prescribed regimens and make lifestyle choices to enhance their health; guard against their patients being inappropriately served or underserved by the health care system; maintain patients' dignity; and ease suffering at the end of life. Yet, as Mathy Mezey and Claire Fagin make clear, the same market-driven forces that make it difficult for physicians to be caring, particularly downsizing and cutbacks in nursing staff, have made it more and more difficult for the nursing profession to make patients its primary concern and to fulfill patients' needs for caring. Moreover, these difficulties create major ethical dilemmas for nurses with respect to their caring responsibilities, such as providing care in unsafe environments, being unable to influence the system on behalf of the patient's need for caring, and redressing systemwide errors in patient care. Mezey and Fagin call for health care institutions to restore a vision that values care and the caregivers charged with assuring a caring environment. To that end, they recommend that hospitals and nursing homes expand the mandates of their ethics committees so that they can become platforms for discussion of the ethical dilemmas of caring in these institutions.

Extended or long-term home- and community-based care for chronically ill and disabled persons of all ages has been taking place for centuries, but in recent decades it has come to the fore as a societal issue because increased longevity has greatly increased the frail elderly population. Although nursing homes have proliferated, fueled by government financing, younger disabled and elderly Americans do not perceive them to be caring environments. The vast majority of people with functionally disabling conditions receive long-term care in their own homes or in other community-based settings, most of it provided on an unpaid, informal basis by family members, friends, and others. As Robyn Stone notes, however, family care is not always caring. It is often filled with conflict and tension, even under the best of circumstances. Long-standing family conflicts may be exacerbated in caregiving situations. Elder abuse and neglect by a family caregiver is far from uncommon; it may not be intentional, but due to stress, ignorance, apathy, or the caregiver's own frailty.

Despite evidence to the contrary, a steadfast belief by public officials in the cost effectiveness of noninstitutional long-term care has led to a shift toward formal, paid caregiving services in the home and other community settings, financed by public funds. The professionalization of home- and community-based care has given rise to institutional structures and controls that often undermine the norms of caring. For example, home care agencies advise their employees not to get too emotionally attached to their clients. And although home care workers recognize the importance of emotional and relational activities, they describe these elements of caring as "outside the job," or "nonwork." As Stone concludes, the caring dimension has been lost in the evolution of home- and community-based care from a private family or neighborhood activity to a formal enterprise with standards, regulations, and profit. She urges formal training requirements for both professional and paraprofessional workers in order to reintroduce the caring dimension, and the provision of monetary and spiritual rewards to motivate workers to engage in the relational aspects of care.

A great deal of effort at caring is undertaken by communities and voluntary organizations, structures that enable communities (both geographically based ones and the nongeographically based) to sustain common interests, goals, and a sense of shared identity. Although there is little systematic research that has evaluated such efforts, four types of organizations and communities that view caring as a central part of their mission appear to have had success in this arena—religious groups; one-on-one programs such as Big Brothers and Big Sisters; support groups (e.g., for cancer patients or cancer survivors, and for caregivers of individuals with Alzheimer disease); and small homogeneous communities (although these can sometimes be oppressive as well as caring).

From an analysis of caring by voluntary organizations, Linda George concludes that their greatest strengths are their flexibility and their ability to develop their own agendas, without the constraints faced by formal service programs of community organizations. Moreover, because of their flexibility, they can make the development of caring relationships their first priority, with specific services being a means to that end. On the other hand, two major obstacles threaten the ability of voluntary organizations to foster caring relationships. First, institutionalization often forces processes of bureaucratization that rival those of other organizations and may require the organization to devote most of its effort to its own survival rather than to serving others. Second, it is not clear that members of voluntary organizations understand what makes their programs acceptable and valued by receivers of caring and their families. Too often, George warns, what is intended as caring ends up imposing the carer's values and agenda on the person in need. A truly caring community, organization, or person will not smother the values of others or fail to respect an individual's needs as that individual defines them, rather than as others define them. A number of issues require research to enable us to understand better the strengths and weaknesses of communities and voluntary organizations as they undertake caring. Yet, as George contends, we do not have to wait for the research evidence to begin to educate the public about caring and to encourage individuals and organizations to commit themselves to it.

How can the success of efforts at caring be appraised? Almost all of the existing procedures for assessing "quality of care" are aimed at curing, not caring. Moreover, as Alvan Feinstein's critical analysis makes clear, the different methods that are commonly used to evaluate quality of care have many flaws. He proposes a new approach for achieving measurements and standards for caring. It begins with open-ended questions addressed to persons who are intimately familiar with what occurs in terms of the needs and activities of caring—patients, family members and other caregivers, and associated contributors—rather than more-distant medical personnel. The answers recorded should not be generalities such as "Thoughtless" or "Communicates well," but should be specific descriptions such as "Abandoned me in the hall outside the radiology suite" or "Told me exactly what to expect when I went for the MRI." When enough specific examples are accumulated, they can be organized into the more general categories of an appropriate taxonomy. In turn, this may lead to a multiple-item inventory, and the performance of the individual cited (e.g., the doctor, nurse, administrator, nurses' aide, visiting nurse, physical or occupational therapist, social worker, clergyperson, family member, close friend, or volunteer) can be given binary ratings such as *yes/no* or *present/absent.* The results can then be used to denote individual problems that need solutions. In addition, the inventory itself can offer details of phenomena to be considered when caring is taught or evaluated. When all the pertinent elements of caring have been identified, the criteria for "successful caring" should be established by the pertinent recipients and participants. As Feinstein emphasizes, they are the most appropriate persons for determining what is needed and wanted and for appraising how well the hopes and desires are fulfilled.

The nature, extent, and quality of caring for individuals are shaped to some extent by the larger societal context within which we live. As a number of chapters in this volume make clear, for example, the organization and financing of health care presently has a negative effect on the capacity of the health professions to be caring. Overall, are we a caring society, as expressed by our governmental actions and inactions with respect to the health of our people? It would be easy enough to assert that the United States is not a caring society, by simply pointing to the fact that at the end of the twentieth century more than 16 percent of Americans had no health insurance while almost every other industrialized nation used the

power of government to assure virtually universal access tc
the situation is much more complex. As Robert Binstock
realistic to evaluate America's governmental approach to h
care by comparing our situation with those of other natioı
stantially different political traditions that are more coll
than ours. His assessment is framed by a delineation of
characteristics of the U.S. political tradition, which reifi
and the free market and militates against governmental ac

Within this context, the extent of governmental a
remarkable—in public health efforts, financing for bioı
and training of health care professionals, and regulatio
providers, insurance companies, and health product ma
distributors. Moreover, even though we rely heavily on th
provide access to health care through employer-sponsorec
ernment has stepped in to provide public insurance—th
Medicaid, and other programs—for selected groups that
cally legitimized as deserving because of "market failure."
count for 46 percent of national health expenditures, anc
ernmental subsidization of employer-sponsored insura
than $100 billion, annually.

Overall, Binstock asserts, there is an incremental trajec
caring as expressed through governmental action, and he
it will be maintained. A number of specific forces will co
new health-related issues to the fore. National voluntary
advocacy groups have become a major force in the ge
health-related issues for the public agenda and are politi
and effective. Their policy agendas are constantly fuelec
ingly sophisticated capacities to monitor health statu
health care; by a burgeoning industry of biological resea
trials, and epidemiological studies; and by questions of fa
generated by technological and biomedical discoveries. Ir
ing health-related issues remain on the agenda for gover
Not the least of these is the matter of insuring the uninsu
challenge would enable all Americans to have access to h
the contributors to this volume hope will become more
today.

INDEX